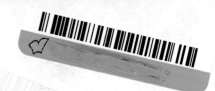

# Neurons *in* Action

## Tutorials and Simulations Using NEURON

*Version 2*

**John W. Moore and Ann E. Stuart**

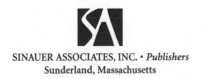

SINAUER ASSOCIATES, INC. • *Publishers*
Sunderland, Massachusetts

*Neurons in Action, Tutorials and Simulations Using NEURON, Version 2*

Address editorial correspondence to:
Sinauer Associates, Inc.
23 Plumtree Road
Sunderland, MA 01375
U.S.A.
Phone: (413) 549-4300
Fax: (413) 549-1118
email: publish@sinauer.com
www.sinauer.com


ISBN 978-0-87893-548-2


Printed in U.S.A.

10 9 8

*Once again to you, Jonathan, our irrepressibly cheerful and devoted colleague and teacher. Your sense of design imbues this version and your superb computer and graphics skills made it happen.*

# Preface

**Our purpose in writing** *Neurons in Action* has been to provide students with tools with which they can appreciate the complexity of the functioning of a single neuron. Students can perform unlimited virtual experiments on digital neurons to test and strengthen their understanding of neurophysiology.

The foundation of the tutorials of *Neurons in Action* is the simulator NEURON, built around the extraordinary set of equations developed by Sir Alan Hodgkin and Sir Andrew Huxley in the 1950's to describe the results of their monumental experiments on the squid's giant axon. These equations remain the reference standard for describing the behavior of excitable membranes. Their unparalleled accuracy allows computer simulations to predict nerve function under the wide variety of circumstances encompassed by these tutorials. Thus, the simulations in *Neurons in Action* reproduce the results of real experiments with remarkable fidelity.

We have included an historical account of the conceptual, technical, experimental, and computational breakthroughs of these pioneers; we are grateful for constructive criticisms and verification of its accuracy by both Hodgkin and Huxley. We are particularly appreciative of the permission to reproduce their papers on the *Neurons in Action* CD granted by Sir Andrew Huxley and the late Sir Alan Hodgkin's family.

We are grateful for the generous support of the National Science Foundation through their Course, Curriculum, and Laboratory Improvement (CCLI) Program, Award Number 0442748. This award made Version 2 possible.

# Contents

# Installation Instructions

*Neurons in Action 2* contains text pages written in HTML, a Firefox browser, and the NEURON software for running simulations. The Firefox browser included with *Neurons in Action* has its own separate preferences that will not interfere with any previous copy of Firefox installed on your computer.

## MAC OS X INSTALLATION

The *Neurons in Action* application contains a universal binary for the NEURON simulation program. Therefore, it will run on both PowerPCs (G3, G4, G5) and Intel Macs.

To install *Neurons in Action 2* on a Mac OS X computer, follow these steps:

1. Insert the *Neurons in Action 2* CD and double-click the CD icon to open it.

2. Open the "NIA2_OSX" folder, and drag the "NIA2 app" icon
    into your Applications folder.

3. After the files have been copied into the Applications folder, eject the CD and then double-click the "NIA2.app" icon that is now in your Applications folder to launch the program.

4. The Firefox browser will be launched, and the *Neurons in Action* homepage will be displayed.

5. If, instead, you see a Firefox update page, simply close the 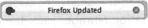 tab to view the *Neurons in Action 2* homepage.

## WINDOWS INSTALLATION

To install *Neurons in Action 2* on a Windows computer, follow these steps:

1. Insert the *Neurons in Action 2* CD. Go to "My Computer" and open the NIA2 CD.

2. Open the "NIA2_Windows" folder, and drag the entire "NIA2PC" folder into your C: drive. (Or Copy the folder and Paste it into your C: drive.)

   **IMPORTANT:** Neurons in Action *will only work when the "NIA2PC" folder is on the C: drive, at the top level, and nowhere else. (**Do not put it into any other folder, such as "Program Files," or on the Desktop.**)*

3. After the files have been copied, eject the CD and then double-click the "NIA2PC" folder that is now in your C: drive to open it.

4. In this folder, double-click the "NIA2PC" program icon to launch *Neurons in Action*.

- If Firefox is already installed on your computer, it will launch and display the *Neurons in Action 2* homepage.

- If Firefox is not already installed on your computer:

  - You will see a message requesting that you allow it to be installed from the installer inside the NIA2 folder. This will be followed by several steps during the installation process. At each step, you may simply click Next to accept the defaults: Setup, License Agreement, Setup Type, Components, Completed.

  - Once the installation is complete, ***Firefox must be closed.***

  - Again click on the "NIA2PC" program icon to launch *Neurons in Action*, and the *Neurons in Action 2* homepage will be displayed.

    (This installation will place a Firefox icon on your desktop, which may be used to launch a personal browser whose bookmarks will not interfere with those of *Neurons in Action*.)

## IMPORTANT NOTE FOR BOTH MAC AND PC

After any future Firefox update is installed (which may happen automatically), or when *Neurons in Action 2* is first launched, the browser may initially display a Firefox update page, instead of the *Neurons in Action 2* homepage.

Close the [ ●     Firefox Updated     ⊗ ] tab to display the *Neurons in Action 2* homepage.

## PROGRAM REGISTRATION

To register your copy of *Neurons in Action 2*, please visit the online registration page: http://www.sinauer.com/nia2

Clicking the "Register" link on the *Neurons in Action* homepage or Bookmarks Bar will also take you to the online registration page. In order to register, you will need the Registration Number from the inside front cover of this manual.

Benefits of registering include receiving information about new versions of *Neurons in Action* and access to free program updates. Registration information will only be used to contact you with information about *Neurons in Action*. Your name and contact information will not be given to anyone else for any other purpose.

## TECHNICAL SUPPORT

For help with installing, running, or registering your copy of *Neurons in Action 2*, please contact Sinauer Associates technical support:

email: support@sinauer.com

Phone: (413) 549-4300

For answers to frequently asked questions and for other useful information, please visit the *Neurons in Action* website: http://www.neuronsinaction.com/

# *Layout of the* Neurons in Action 2 *Interface*

When you click on a tutorial, here is the interface you will see. The graphics below lead you through the structure of this interface so that you can be aware of your options, particularly the content of the expandable menus.

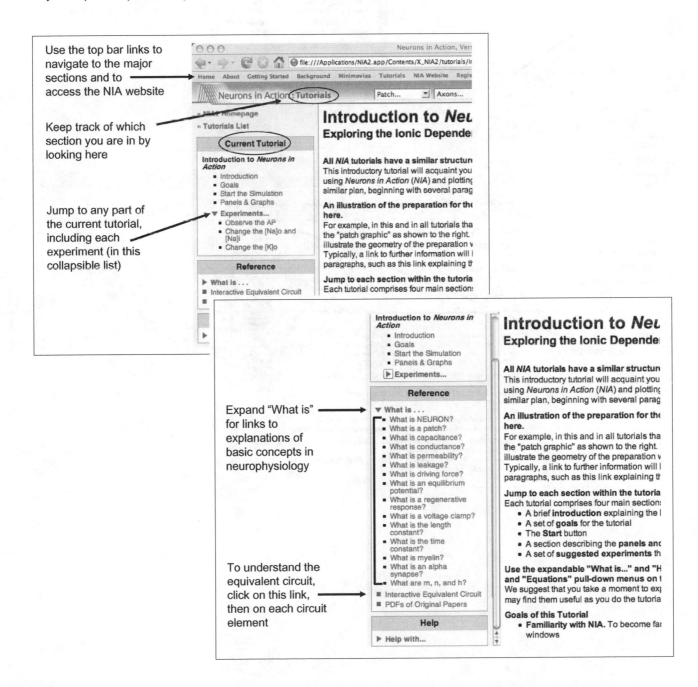

Expand the "Help with" section....

...then expand each individual Help item

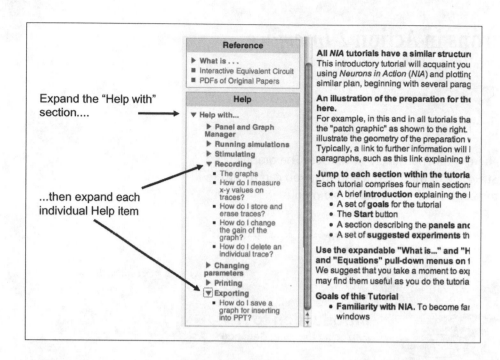

Pull down each of these three menus to access links to the tutorials by geometry: Patch, Axons, Cells

Pull down each of these two menus to access links to History topics or Equations (as shown).

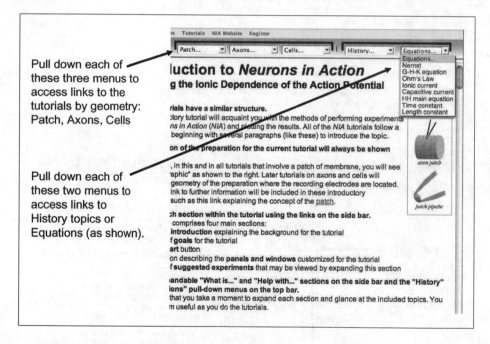

# Layout of the Panels and Graphs

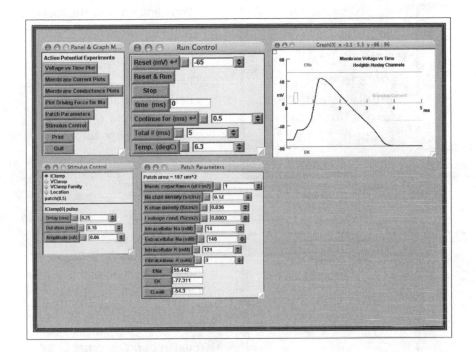

### Basic layout of the panels and graphs

The panels and graphs of *NIA* are placed on the computer screen in certain positions that are the same from tutorial to tutorial. Here is the basic layout of the screen.

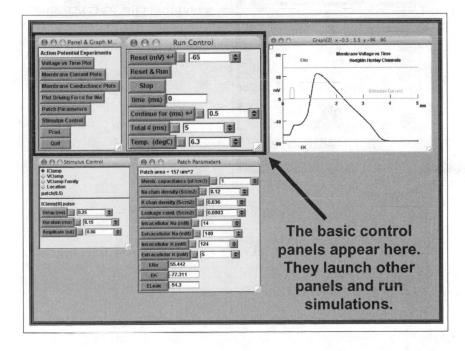

The basic control panels appear here. They launch other panels and run simulations.

### Upper left quadrant

- The Panel and Graph (P&G) Manager (left) has buttons to call up other panels and to quit the simulation.
- The Run Control panel (right) runs, stops, and pauses simulations. You can change the starting "Reset" voltage (the resting potential) and the temperature.

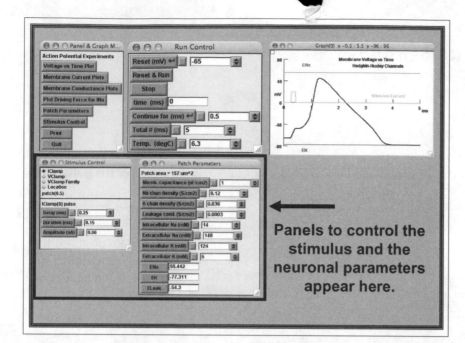

**Panels to control the stimulus and the neuronal parameters appear here.**

**Lower left quadrant**

- In the Stimulus Control panel (left) you choose whether to stimulate the preparation with current (IClamp) or control the voltage (VClamp and VClampFamily). You specify the pulse parameters. You can also view the location of your stimulating electrode.

- In the Patch Parameters Panel (right), you can change neuronal parameters or ion concentration. This menu differs from one tutorial to the next.

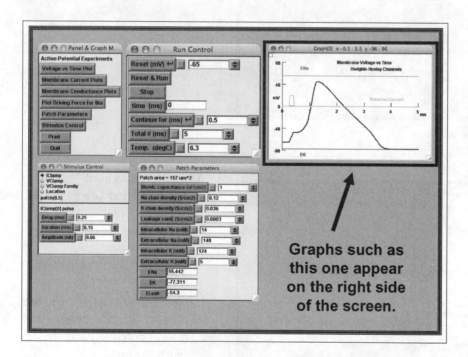

**Graphs such as this one appear on the right side of the screen.**

**Right half of screen**

The Voltage-vs-Time Graph, shown here, typifies the graphs that appear on the right side of the screen when you launch the simulation.

You can bring up other graphs in this space by clicking their buttons in the P&G Manager. The particular graphs available for launching depend on the tutorial.

# *Introduction to* Neurons in Action

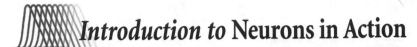

## Exploring the Ionic Dependence of the Action Potential

**All *NIA* tutorials have a similar structure.**
This introductory tutorial will acquaint you with the methods of performing experiments using *Neurons in Action* (*NIA*) and plotting the results. All of the *NIA* tutorials follow a similar plan, beginning with several paragraphs (like these) to introduce the topic.

**An illustration of the preparation for the current tutorial will always be shown here.**
For example, in this and in all tutorials that involve a patch of membrane, you will see the "patch graphic" as shown to the right. Later tutorials on axons and cells will illustrate the geometry of the preparation where the recording electrodes are located. Typically, a link to further information will be included in these introductory paragraphs, such as this link explaining the concept of the <u>patch</u>.

**Jump to each section within the tutorial using the links on the side bar.**
Each tutorial comprises four main sections:
- A brief **introduction** explaining the background for the tutorial
- A set of **goals** for the tutorial
- The **Start** button
- A section describing the **panels and windows** customized for the tutorial
- A set of **suggested experiments** that may be viewed by expanding this section

**Use the expandable "What Is..." and "Help with..." sections on the side bar and the "History" and "Equations" pull-down menus on the top bar.**
We suggest that you take a moment to expand each section and glance at the included topics. You may find them useful as you do the tutorials.

### Goals of this Tutorial
- **Familiarity with *NIA*.** To become familiar with the overall layout of the *NIA* panels and graphing windows
- **Stimulating and recording.** To understand how to stimulate your preparation and record the results
- **Experimenting.** To become adept at performing an experiment in *NIA* by changing parameters
- **Observing the action potential.** To reproduce the first key observations of the action potential: its dependence on Na and K ions

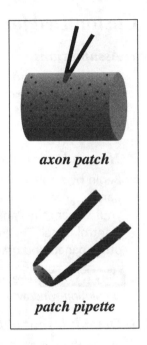

*axon patch*

*patch pipette*

## Start the Simulation

Click this button to bring up the panels and windows of the simulation.

**Start the Simulation**

## Description of the Panels and Windows Customized for this Tutorial

### 1. Assumptions

This tutorial assumes that you are totally unfamiliar with the basic manipulations of *NIA* and explains them in some detail. For more information, consult the descriptions of panels, windows, and manipulations under "Help with..." on the side bar.

### 2. How to launch the "lab" where you can run your simulations

Begin by single-clicking the "Start the Simulation" button. Two "manager panels" that anchor every tutorial will come up in the top-left section of your screen: the Panel and Graph Manager (P&G Manager) and the Run Control panel. The P&G Manager has buttons that allow you to call up other panels and graphs.

**ATTENTION!** *Use Atl-Tab (PC) or Command-Tab (Mac) to toggle between simulation windows and tutorial text.*

### 3. Default layout of the panels and graphs on the screen

In *NIA* there is an overall structure to the appearance of the panels and windows that remains the same from tutorial to tutorial. The details differ, however, from one tutorial to the next. As you bring up the panels and windows in the sequence below, you will discover that they are positioned on the screen in three major sectors:

- **Upper-left sector:** The two "manager panels" always appear here.

- **Lower-left sector:** The panels allowing you to stimulate the preparation and control experimental parameters will appear here.

- **Right side of screen:** All of the graphs will appear here.

### 4. Managing your simulations

- <u>**Panel & Graph Manager:**</u> In this panel, buttons specific for each tutorial allow you to call up graphs or windows. In the present tutorial, the P&G Manager has only five buttons; later ones typically have more.

  - **Click Stimulus Control:** This button launches the panel in which you will control the stimulus pulse to be delivered to your preparation. Calling up this panel is like inserting a stimulating electrode into a cell.

  - **Click Voltage-vs-Time Plot:** This button launches a graph where you will observe the voltage response to a stimulus.

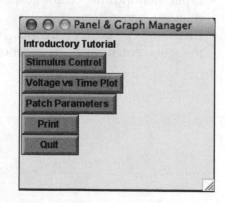

- **Click Patch Parameters:** This button launches a panel (lower-left sector) where you can perform experiments on your preparation by changing the parameters such as ion concentration or channel density.

- **Print:** This button calls up a panel allowing you to print your results. Specific instructions for "Printing" may be found under "Help with..." in the side bar.

- **Quit:** This button ends the simulation and closes all of the panels and graphs.

- **Run Control:** This panel always appears just to the right of the P&G Manager. It triggers and controls the running of the simulations: the value of the potential at the start of the simulation, the duration of the simulation, and the temperature. In this panel you can also pause a simulation or inch it along a time or space axis. Experiment with these buttons as you need them: Simply refer back to this section as necessary.

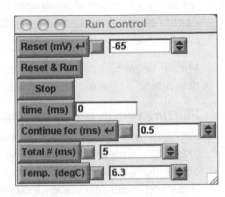

  - **Reset (mV):** The value in the white field is the initial potential of the patch, axon, or cell at the start of the simulation. Think of it as the resting potential. NEURON calculates the values of the initial conductances for this voltage. You may change it, and then NEURON will calculate new initial conductances.

  - **Reset & Run (R&R):** Clicking this button resets the initial conditions ($t = 0$ and initial voltage and conductances) and starts a simulation.

  - **Stop:** This button stops the simulation.

  - **Time (ms):** The field associated with this button shows physiological time as the simulation progresses.

  - **Continue for (ms):** This button allows you to run the simulation in a pause-advance mode. Each click on this button, after you have "Reset," allows you to continue the run for the interval of time shown in the white field.

  - **Total # (ms):** This button simultaneously sets the duration of the run and the time scale in the graph(s) displaying the results of the simulation.

  - **Temp. (degC):** Here you can set the temperature for the simulation.

## 5. *Stimulating your preparation*

- **Stimulus Control, "Location" selected:** When you insert a stimulating electrode into the patch (by clicking the Stimulus Control button in the P&G Manager), the location of the stimulating electrode is selected by default. The electrode (blue dot) is positioned on a line representing the preparation (a patch in this tutorial). Here the microelectrode is in the middle (0.5 position) of a patch, indicated by "patch(0.5)" under the word "Location" in the upper panel. (You can think of the patch as a tiny portion of an axon or as a piece of membrane sealed across the opening of a "patch pipette.")

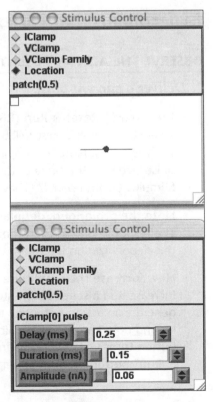

- **Stimulus Control, "IClamp" selected:** When you select "IClamp" (current clamp), the parameters of the stimulus pulse will be displayed in the lower panel. Use these default parameters to begin your set of experiments. You can change any of these settings by using the <u>Arrows Box</u> to the right of the white field or by placing your cursor in the field and typing a new value.

**PLEASE NOTE!**

*PC: Once you have selected a panel, single-click on a button. Double-clicking will bring up the panel or window twice. If you accidentally launch two Stimulus Control panels, for example, you will insert not one but two electrodes into the patch, which may lead to puzzling results.*

*Mac: A single click on a panel or button will notify the simulator that it should now attend to the button's actions. Then the instructions above apply.*

6. *Plotting your results on a Voltage-vs-Time graph*

   Click the "Voltage vs Time Plot" button in the P&G Manager. A specific <u>graphical window</u> for plotting membrane potential versus time will appear on the right-hand portion of the screen. Think of launching this window as "inserting" your recording electrode "into" the patch.

7. *Doing an experiment using the <u>Patch Parameters</u> panel*

   Now click the "Patch Parameters" button in the P&G Manager. In the panel that comes up you will see the starting (default) concentrations for Na and K outside and inside the cell. In the "Experiments and Observations" section below, you will change these concentrations, re-run the simulation, and observe what happens to the action potential.

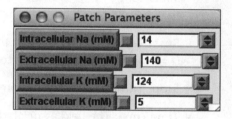

# Experiments and Observations

## OBSERVE THE ACTION POTENTIAL

1. *Deliver a current pulse*

   - **Press (click) Reset & Run (R&R) in the Run Control panel.**
     A very brief current pulse will be displayed as the green trace on the Voltage-vs-Time graph. Note the amplitude, delay, and duration of the current pulse. Are they the same as the values specified in your IClamp in the Stimulus Control panel? (They had better be.)

   - **Note the prolonged, depolarizing voltage response.**
     The response is long even though the stimulating current is brief. Why this depolarization lasts so long is explored in the <u>Threshold</u> tutorial.

   - **Now increase the amplitude of the stimulating current.**
     Increase it in a series of tiny steps to see if you can stimulate this patch to generate an action potential. Increase the amplitude either by using the <u>up and down arrows</u> or by clicking your cursor in the white field (the button turns yellow) and typing in a number. When you click the "Reset & Run" button (R&R), the default value changes and a red square (or

checkmark) appears in the box associated with the button. (Simply click the red square to restore the default value.) Choose "Keep Lines" from the graph submenu (see below) to save each of your responses.

- **Observe the voltage responses.**
  You have delivered subthreshold and suprathreshold stimuli to your patch. Note that the action potential is an "all or none" event—it is a little explosion that either happens or does not.

- **Measure the peak amplitude of the action potential.**
  The "Crosshair" option in the submenu is selected by default. When you place your cursor anywhere on the action potential trace, the $x$ and $y$ values of the cursor's position will appear in the top bar of the graph.

**SUBMENU FOR PLOTTING OPTIONS** *To bring up these menus, make sure your cursor is on the plotting window and then click the right mouse button. Mac users can also click the little square in the upper-left corner of the graph. The left menu comes up first; by sliding your cursor to "View" the right-hand submenu appears. Useful options at this point include "Keep Lines," "Erase," and the default setting "Crosshair," indicated by the black diamond. "View = plot" will adjust the gain of the plot so that the trace fills it.*

| View . . . | View = plot |
| --- | --- |
| Crosshair | Set View |
| Plot what? | 10% Zoom out |
| Color/Brush | 10% Zoom in |
| Axis Type | NewView |
| Keep Lines | Zoom in/out |
| Erase | Translate |
| Move Text | Round View |
| Change Text | Whole Scene |
| Delete | Scene=View |
| | Object Name |

## 2. *Observe the duration of the undershoot and the return of the voltage to rest*

- **Increase the running time of the simulation.**
  Using "Total # (ms)" in Run Control, increase the time to 10 ms. If you type the value into the white field, your cursor must be located within the field. Alternatively you can click the "up" arrow in the Arrows Box.

- **Notice how long the voltage takes to return to the resting level.**
  Following the action potential, the membrane is completely inexcitable (refractory); it slowly recovers its excitability as the voltage returns to its resting value. In the Na Action Potential tutorial you will explore this period of refractoriness.

## 3. *Change the temperature*

- **Increase and decrease the temperature in the Run Control panel**
  To compare the action potentials at different temperatures, use "Keep Lines." Notice the main changes in the action potential as you increase or decrease the temperature. Later tutorials will focus on the effects of temperature on action potential threshold and propagation.

### DO EXPERIMENTS: CHANGE THE EXTRACELLULAR Na CONCENTRATION, [Na]o, AND THEN THE INTRACELLULAR Na CONCENTRATION, [Na]i

You can reproduce the classic experiments of Hodgkin and Katz (1949) on squid giant axons. They found that the amplitude and rate of rise of the action potential were highly dependent on the [Na]o. Furthermore, you can also do an experiment for which the techniques were not available at the time: You can change the [Na]i.

### 1. First change the [Na]o: How does the action potential change?

- **Start by eliciting an action potential in normal [Na]o.**
  Set the amplitude of your current to a value that will elicit an action potential. Choose "Keep Lines" from the submenu on the Voltage-vs-Time graph so that you can save the family of action potentials you are about to plot.

- **Now change the [Na]o and observe the action potential.**
  In the Patch Parameters panel, change the [Na]o from its default value of 140 mM to higher and lower values. Make your changes over a wide range (e.g., by two fold steps) from double the default value down to a value equal to the internal concentration.

  (If you are familiar with underlying equilibrium potentials and the Nernst equation, plot the peak of the action potential and ENa as a function of [Na]o. You can check your plot of ENa versus [Na]o against ours.)

  You must have observed that during the action potential the membrane voltage actually reverses sign and the membrane becomes transiently positive inside. This observation, along with knowing that the [Na]i is typically very low, and the membrane is not permeable to Na at rest, led Andrew Huxley and Alan Hodgkin to postulate that during the action potential the membrane becomes selectively permeable to Na ions.

### 2. Compare your simulated results with classic observations

- **You can compare your results to those in the PDF of the original paper.**
  Throughout the *NIA* tutorials you will have a chance to compare your results with published observations by clicking hyperlinks to original papers. Hodgkin and Katz (1949) tested Hodgkin and Huxley's Na hypothesis. In their paper, how did the amplitude (their Figures 4 and 8) and rate of rise (their Figure 10) of the action potential depend on the Na concentration? The introduction section of this paper clearly lays out the thinking of these brilliant scientists about this important problem—the mechanism of the action potential—and is well worth reading.

- **By how much can you reduce the [Na]o and still get an action potential?**
  Does this value surprise you? The action potential has a huge "safety factor"; that is, even if the [Na]o changes quite a bit, the action potential will still occur. This is worth keeping in mind in considering pathological situations where the [Na] in the blood is too high or too low.

  The Equilibrium Potentials and Na Action Potential tutorials should give you more insight into the mechanism of the action potential.

- **Return [Na]o to its default value.**
  To do this, click the box associated with the "Extracellular Na (mM)" button. The box contains a red square when you change its value; the red square disappears when you click the box back to the default value.

### 3. Now change the [Na]i: How does the action potential change?
Go beyond what Hodgkin and Katz were able to do and perfuse the axon internally with a solution of your choice. (Later, this experiment was done by

squeezing out the axon's cytoplasm and replacing it with saline.) You can mimic a "very tired nerve" experiment by doubling the [Na]i and then repeating changes in the [Na]o. How should the plots change if the [Na]i is doubled?

- **Experiment with changing the [Na]i.**
  (In a real experiment this would be very difficult.) What happens if you set the [Na]i to the same value as the [Na]o? Do you get the same result as when you set the [Na]o to the same value as the [Na]i? Keep these observations in mind when you do the Equilibrium Potentials and Na Action Potential tutorials.

## EXPERIMENT WITH THE [K]o

### 1. Increase the [K]o

- **How does the action potential change?**
  First make sure that your [Na]o and [Na]i are returned to their default values by clicking the box associated with their buttons. Now (1) "Erase" whatever is on your graph, (2) choose "Keep Lines," (3) increase the [K]o in several steps, and (4) observe what happens to the action potential.

- **Make a huge change in concentration.**
  If this were an experiment on a live preparation, you could not do the following outrageous experiment: What happens if you *really* increase [K]o, say to 2000 mM? From both of these experiments, what part of the action potential do you conclude depends on the [K]? Note that in *NIA*, all experiments start at the initial potential specified in the Run Control panel ("Reset (mv)" button) regardless of what ion concentration you have chosen; the concentration is essentially changed at the start of the simulation.

  You will find out in the Equilibrium Potentials tutorial that changing the [K]o by even a small amount alters the resting potential and the excitability of a membrane.

## NOW PRESS "QUIT" AND GO TO THE NEXT TUTORIAL

If you feel comfortable with these basic manipulations of *NIA*, press the "Quit" button in the P&G Manager. Then click the "Yes" button to affirm that you really want to quit.

**PLEASE NOTE!** *You must quit each simulation before going to the next one to avoid having multiple copies of NEURON running, each with a different simulation and set of panels, electrodes, and settings.*

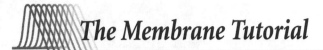

# The Membrane Tutorial

## How Currents Depolarize Excitable Membranes

**Here, you will build an excitable membrane.**
How do the component parts of membranes (the capacitance of the lipids, the pumps, and the conductances of the channels) work together to permit voltage signaling? The simulations below approach this question by starting with a bare lipid bilayer membrane and adding new mechanisms in a stepwise fashion.

**You will inject current across the membrane and measure the resulting change in the voltage.**
You will deliver a pulse of current across the membrane and observe how it changes the voltage across the <u>capacitance of the membrane</u>. Further, you will observe the capacitive current flowing onto the membrane during the pulse. These experiments are carried out in a "<u>patch</u>."

**Goals of this Tutorial**
- To understand, through experimentation, how a current pulse changes the voltage across a membrane:
  - When it is only a plain lipid bilayer
  - When it has only a Na/K pump that establishes a resting potential
  - When it has, in addition to the pump, a voltage-insensitive, nonselective "leakage" conductance
  - When it has, in addition to the pump and leakage channels, the voltage-sensitive Na and K channels described by Hodgkin and Huxley
- To understand capacitance and capacitive currents and why they are important for understanding neuronal signaling

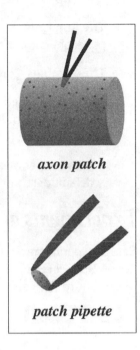

*axon patch*

*patch pipette*

## Start the Simulation

Click this button to bring up the panels and windows of the simulation.

> **Start the Simulation**

## Description of the Panels and Windows Customized for this Tutorial

### 1. Assumptions

We assume you have worked through the <u>Introduction</u> to *Neurons in Action* tutorial and are familiar with the general structure of the simulation panels. Here we describe the panels and graphs, customized for the Membrane Tutorial.

## 2. *Starting the simulation, three panels appear*

- **The P&G Manager, in the upper-left corner**

  - The upper four buttons bring up graphs one by one linked to the experiments below; they will lie on top of one another as they are called up.

  - The "Capacitive Current vs Time" and "Membrane Parameters" buttons call up windows that will be useful later in the tutorial.

- **The Run Control panel, next to the P&G Manager.** The buttons on this panel are common to all of the tutorials.

- **The Stimulus Control panel, below the other two panels.**

  - When launched, this panel automatically inserts a stimulating electrode into the patch. By default, the "Location" option is selected, showing the electrode (blue ball) located in the center of the patch (the line).

  - In the experiments below, you will click the IClamp diamond to see the default delay, duration, and amplitude of the stimulus current pulse.

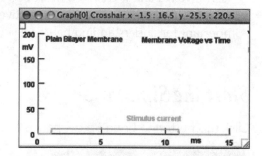

# *Experiments and Observations*

Before experimenting, please read here about capacitance, electrical "equivalent circuits," and why the concept of capacitance is useful and important to the neuroscientist.

**PLEASE NOTE!** *In The Membrane Tutorial it is important to bring up the panels in the prescribed sequence in order to avoid confusing NEURON.*

### EXPERIMENT WITH CHARGING A LIPID BILAYER WITH A CURRENT PULSE

## 1. *First, observe how a current pulse charges a membrane*

- **Press the "Plain Bilayer Membrane" button (in the P&G Manager) to call up a Voltage-vs-Time graph.**
  In this simplest possible experiment you will deliver a current pulse to the membrane and observe the rate of change of the voltage across the membrane capacitance (as represented by the circuit illustration below). Note that depolarizations will be plotted from zero: As yet, there is no resting potential in this cell.

- **Run the simulation: Charge the membrane.**
  When you press the "Reset & Run" button in the Run Control panel, the stimulating electrode will deliver the current pulse to the membrane and the voltage across the membrane will be plotted. The plotted current pulse has no associated scale but is proportional to the stimulus current. Observe that the membrane potential changes as a linear ramp until the current ceases; from that time forth the

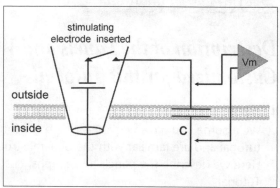

voltage stays at that level. The membrane is charged to a certain voltage; it will stay at this voltage since there is no path for the current to leave the capacitor.

- **Press the "Capacitive Current vs Time" button to call up a second graph.**
  This graph will appear beneath the Voltage-vs-Time graph and will show the capacitive current density (capacitive current per unit area) being plotted when you run a simulation.

  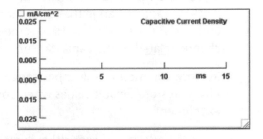

  Note that the amplitude of the stimulus current pulse is 2 nA, and the area of the patch is 0.0001 cm$^2$ (displayed on the Membrane Parameters panel). Thus the capacitive current density across the plain lipid bilayer will be 0.02 mA/cm$^2$.

- **Calculate the *expected* rate of change of membrane voltage from the equation for capacitive current.**
  You can measure the rate of change of the voltage to see if it agrees with your calculation. Consult this link if you need assistance.

- **Store your traces for comparison with the next experimental result.**
  To save a plot for comparison with a new plot when you make changes below, use the "Keep Lines" feature. Place your cursor in the plotting window, click the right mouse button, hold it down, and then select this option. The cursor *must* be placed within the plotting window for this option to work. (Macs: click on the tiny box in the upper-left corner of the graph.) If you right-click again and view the submenu, you will see a red check next to "Keep Lines," confirming your selection.

## 2. Change the amplitude of the current pulse

- **Press the "IClamp" diamond in the Stimulus Control panel.**
  The parameters of the current pulse will be revealed in the lower half of the panel. Change the current stimulus amplitude with the arrows to the right of the white value field or with the field editor. You *must* have the cursor positioned in the white field when you enter changes using the keyboard.

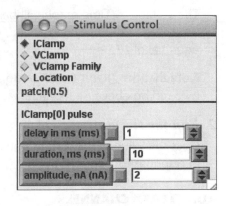

- **Click "Reset & Run" with the amplitude at its new value.**
  If the plot axes are too large or need expansion, you can resize them by right-clicking on the graph and selecting View = plot. If you wish to restore the original size, however, you will have to first close and then re-open the graphing window.

  Is the slope of the voltage change directly proportional to the current amplitude? Should it be? Click this link if you are unsure.

- **Erase your plots and restore the default current setting to prepare for the next experiment.**
  You can clear the plot at any time with the "Erase" feature in the menu called up by the right mouse button. You can restore the default setting by clicking on the box with the red mark on it.

### 3. Change the membrane capacitance

- **Call up the Membrane Parameters panel.**
  If you have not already done so, press that button in the
  P&G Manager. Change the capacitance, click "Keep Lines,"
  and re-run the simulation. How is the slope of the voltage
  change <u>related</u> to the capacitance?

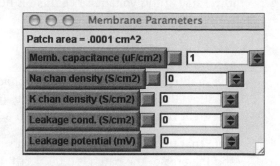

- **Restore the membrane capacitance to its default value.**
  Always restore default values when you are finished with an
  experiment.

- **Do you understand capacitive currents?**
  Understanding <u>capacitive current</u> is the first step in understanding the
  famous <u>Hodgkin-Huxley (HH) equation</u> used throughout the *NIA* tutorials.
  The first term in this equation is the capacitive current: the product of the
  membrane capacitance and the rate of change of the voltage. For the
  plain lipid bilayer, the HH equation is reduced simply to this first term
  because neither a leak conductance nor voltage-sensitive channels are
  included in this basic membrane.

## ESTABLISH A RESTING POTENTIAL BY ADDING THE Na/K PUMP

The resting potential comes about through the action of the <u>Na/K pump</u> (or
Na/K ATPase), which simultaneously moves Na ions out of the cell and K ions
in. How the precise value of the resting potential is achieved is approached in
the <u>Equilibrium Potentials</u> tutorial.

### 1. Press the "Add the Na/K pump" button to establish a resting potential

The Voltage-vs-Time graph will be overlaid by a new one showing that a
simulated pump has been added, charging the membrane to a resting
potential of –75 mV.

Note that the "Reset (mV)" button in the Run Control panel now is marked
by a red box because its value has been changed from 0 to –75 mV.

### 2. Run the simulation

Does the value of the resting potential <u>affect</u> the slope of the voltage ramp
in response to a current pulse?

## ADD "LEAK" CHANNELS

Hodgkin and Huxley observed a voltage-insensitive
(linear) current in the squid axon with a reversal potential
near the resting value. They referred to this current as
"<u>leak</u>" and incorporated it into their <u>equation</u> to make
the net current equal to zero at rest. Here we will place
these very simple "leak" channels into our plain membrane to see how adding a simple resistor affects the
charging and discharging of the lipid bilayer capacitor.
Note in the diagram that, in contrast to the plain lipid
bilayer, there is now a path ($r_{leak}$) for current stored on
the capacitor to leak back out across the membrane.

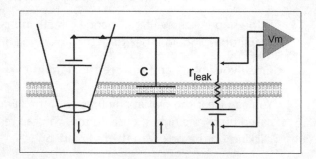

### 1. Press the "Add Leak Channels" button

A new Voltage-vs-Time graph will replace the previous one.

- The value of the "leak" conductance assigned by Hodgkin and Huxley ($0.0003$ S/cm$^2$) now shows up in the "Leakage conductance" field of the Membrane Parameters panel. We replace the mho—the original unit for conductance used in the Hodgkin-Huxley papers—with the present-day notation, the siemens (S).

  - The "Leakage potential" has been set to –70 mV (from its previous value of –75 mV) to reflect the reduction in resting potential upon addition of a leak.

### 2. Run the simulation

Now, the time course of the change in voltage across the membrane is quite different from what you saw for a plain lipid bilayer.

In the Hodgkin-Huxley (HH) equation there are now two terms that describe the situation at this point in the tutorial: the first term (for capacitive current), and the last term (the leak current). The other two terms are still zero because there are as yet no voltage-sensitive channels in the membrane.

### 3. Be quantitative

Measure the amplitude and time constant of the voltage change. These measurements are widely used in neurophysiological experiments.

## ADD HODGKIN-HUXLEY (HH) VOLTAGE-SENSITIVE CHANNELS

Add the HH Na and K channels to the membrane to enable it to generate action potentials upon depolarization.

### 1. Press the "Add HH Channels" button in the P&G Manager

Again, an appropriate Voltage-vs-Time graph will open on top of the previous one. The default values for the densities (proportional to conductances) of the Na and K channels (as well as the HH values for the leak conductance and reversal potential) will appear in the "Membrane Parameters" panel. The resting potential (viewed in the "Reset" field in the Run Control panel) is further reduced by the small leak of Na into the cell. This matter will be further explored in the Equilibrium Potentials tutorial.

### 2. Run the simulation

You should observe that two action potentials are generated during the current pulse. The capacitive current surges at the onset and offset of the pulse as it did in the

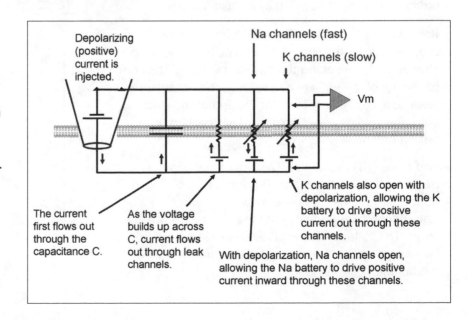

Depolarizing (positive) current is injected.

Na channels (fast)

K channels (slow)

Vm

The current first flows out through the capacitance C.

As the voltage builds up across C, current flows out through leak channels.

With depolarization, Na channels open, allowing the Na battery to drive positive current inward through these channels.

K channels also open with depolarization, allowing the K battery to drive positive current out through these channels.

previous exercise, but during the action potentials it has a <u>more complicated shape</u>. (Remember that you can "turn down the gain" for the capacitive current plot using the "View = plot" option on the pop-up menu. To restore the original gain, close and reopen the window.)

### 3. *Consider these questions*

- Why is the capacitive current so large?

- Do you know at what point in the action potential the capacitive current is at its peak?

- At what point in the action potential does the capacitive current cross zero?

- During the falling phase of the action potential, why is the capacitive current more prolonged but smaller than during the rising phase?

- Click here for <u>answers</u>.

### 4. *Experiment with increasing the duration of the current pulse*

In the Stimulus Control panel, increase the stimulus current duration and then increase the "Total # ms" in the Run Control panel, as you did above. Will spikes <u>continue to be generated</u> at this rate indefinitely?

## Summary

The two composite figures here summarize the three steps of this tutorial carried out with a resting potential. The upper figure shows the voltage responses to the current pulses at low gain; the lower figure shows the first few milliseconds at high gain and expanded time base to enable you to resolve the differences between the traces in this time period.

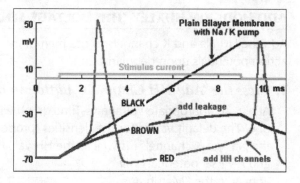

- **Black trace**: When the current pulse charges the bare membrane, the voltage rises as a linear ramp.

- **Brown trace (leakage)**: The addition of leakage channels causes the voltage to deviate from the ramp after an initial rise along the ramp's trajectory. The rate of change of the voltage decreases as the voltage rises towards a steady-state level. At the end of the current pulse the voltage decays exponentially back to the resting potential.

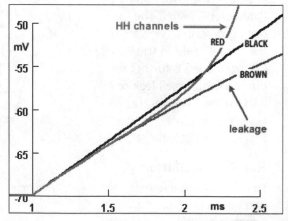

- **Red trace (HH channels)**: The addition of voltage-gated Na and K (HH) channels does not cause a noticeable change (from the voltage rise when only leak channels are present) until the action potential arises. The voltage then explosively increases at a rate far surpassing the linear ramp for the purely capacitive membrane.

In the expanded version of the figure you can see that the red curve initially overlays the brown curve (leakage conductance). This happens because the resting state conductances of the HH channels are insignificant compared to that of the leakage.

## PRESS "QUIT" TO GO TO THE NEXT TUTORIAL

### 1. Press the "Quit" button (in the P&G Manager)

This button terminates the tutorial. It is distinct from "Close," which simply closes a panel.

### 2. Confirm by clicking on the "Yes" button in the dialog box

**ATTENTION!** *You must quit each simulation before going to the next to avoid having multiple copies of NEURON running, each with a different simulation and set of panels, electrodes, and settings.*

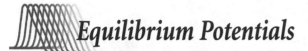

# *Equilibrium Potentials*

## Determinants of Signals and the Resting Potential

**Understanding equilibrium potentials is fundamental to understanding cell signaling and excitability.**
In this tutorial you can experiment with intracellular and extracellular Na and K concentrations to see how they determine ENa and EK, the <u>equilibrium potentials</u> for these ions. You can then vary the ratio between the cell's conductance to K and to Na to understand how ion selectivity determines the membrane potential (Vm). In subsequent tutorials you will see that Vm controls the opening of ion channels and the generation of signals in neurons, skeletal muscle, and heart muscle. Thus, excitability depends ultimately on precisely regulated ionic concentrations.

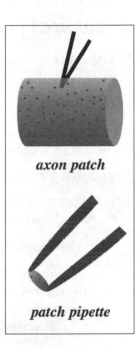

*axon patch*

*patch pipette*

**Equilibrium potentials are calculated, not measured.**
While Vm is a cell property that is observed and measured, Eion is *calculated* by the <u>Nernst equation</u>. The equilibrium potential for an ion (Eion) and the membrane potential (Vm) are equal only under one special circumstance: when the cell is permeable (has conductance) *only* to that ion. Eion depends only on three variables: (1) the ratio of the concentrations of that ion inside and outside of the cell, (2) the absolute temperature (273 degrees + experimental temperature in centigrade), and (3) the valence of the ion.

**If the ion concentrations do not change, ENa and EK do not change.**
Vm can soar from negative to positive values and back again but the equilibrium potentials remain steady at their values. If the cell becomes permeable only to Na ions, then Vm will soar to ENa. If it then becomes permeable only to K ions, Vm will plunge back to EK. In fact, when Na and K are the only ions to consider, Vm is trapped between ENa and EK. Notice how the changes in Vm—changes that ultimately constitute signals—can be generated simply by changing the relative ionic conductances (<u>permeabilities</u>) of the cell with time.

**Conversely, if the extracellular ion concentrations change, then EK or ENa will change, with potentially harmful consequences.**
A change in an equilibrium potential can thus greatly affect the Vm of cells and lead to pathological conditions. For example, a slight increase in the [K] in the blood due to dehydration can have very serious <u>consequences</u>.

**Goals of this Tutorial**
- To understand equilibrium potentials by experimenting with ion concentrations and calculating them using the Nernst equation
- To understand how the resting potential depends on the relative permeabilities (conductances) of Na and K
- To understand how signals can be generated by changing the ratio of the conductances to Na (gNa) and K (gK)

## Start the Simulation

Click this button to bring up the panels and windows of the simulation.

Start the Simulation

## Description of the Panels and Windows Customized for this Tutorial

### 1. The P&G Manager

Three buttons in the P&G Manager bring up specific Voltage-vs-Time plots for patches containing the K conductance only, the Na conductance only, or both. Launching each graph, when called for in the tutorial, is equivalent to inserting a recording electrode into the patch containing the specified conductance. (The graphs appear on top of one another.)

### 2. The Patch Parameters panel

In the Patch Parameters panel, you can change ion concentrations and also the ratio of the Na and K conductances (also referred to as channel densities).

- **Ion channel densities (conductances):**

  - In this tutorial (but not in other tutorials), the values of the Na and K channel densities have been drastically changed from normal so that they can be expressed as ratios. In the other *NIA* tutorials the channel densities will be the actual Hodgkin-Huxley values.

  - Here, and throughout *NIA*, we will treat permeability and conductance as if they are the same property, although this is not strictly true. We will refer to the Na conductance as gNa and to the K conductance as gK.

- **Ionic concentrations:** The default Na and K concentrations are typical for mammals, frogs, and other terrestrial animals.

- **Equilibrium potentials for the ions:** The equilibrium potentials are calculated automatically by the Nernst equation from the Na and K concentrations that are set by default, or by you.

  **ATTENTION!** *Remember to single-click on a button. Double-clicking will bring up the panel or window twice!*

## Experiments and Observations

### EXPERIMENT WITH A GLIAL CELL, WHICH IS SOLELY PERMEABLE TO K IONS

Many glial cells are permeable only to K ions; they have no measurable Na permeability. Because of this, the glial Vm acts as a "K electrode"—that is, its resting membrane potential will always be equal to its calculated EK. Long ago, Steve Kuffler realized this and used the Vm of glial cells to report the value of the [K] in the extracellular spaces of the leech CNS when neurons fired trains of action potentials (Kuffler and Nicholls 1966).

### 1. Press the "K Conductance Only" button (P&G Manager) to mimic a patch from a glial cell

A Voltage-vs-Time graph will appear. In the Patch Parameters panel, note that the Na channel density, or conductance (gNa), is automatically set to zero. The K channel density (gK) is set to one. The choice of one is arbitrary and not the actual value of gK in a normal axon, since we will be simply looking at conductance ratios in this tutorial. Should this <u>matter to our calculation</u> of EK?

### 2. To record Vm, run the simulation

Click the "Run" button on the <u>Run Control panel</u>. In the Membrane Voltage-vs-Time plot you will see a blue horizontal line—the glial resting potential. Measure its value with the crosshairs. Because the glial cell is only permeable to K, Vm should equal EK. Check this by comparing your <u>crosshairs</u> measurement to the value of EK in the Patch Parameters panel. From now on, blue will be the color of the EK line.

### 3. Change the [K]o (extracellular [K])

In the Patch Parameters panel, change the [K]o from its default value of 5 mM to higher and lower values. Each time you change the concentration and click Run, you will see that EK changes: The simulator NEURON is using the <u>Nernst equation</u> to calculate the value of EK for you from the logarithm of the ratio of [K]o to [K]i (extracellular to intracellular [K]).

### 4. Plot EK versus [K]o.

Your plot should be similar to the upper figure shown in <u>this link</u>.

### 5. <u>Questions</u> to test your understanding of the Nernst equation

- What value of [K]o will cause EK to be exactly zero and why?

- If the [K] values were reversed such that [K]o = 124 and [K]i = 5 mM, what would be the value of EK?

- For the same values of [K]o and [K]i, will EK be different in a mammal than in these simulations?

## WHAT WOULD HAPPEN TO Vm IF THE MEMBRANE WERE TO BECOME PERMEABLE ONLY TO Na IONS?

### 1. Press the "Na conductance only" button

A new graph will open on top of the previous one. In the Patch Parameters panel you will see that the Na conductance is reset to one and that the K conductance is set to zero.

### 2. Run the simulation

Now, because the membrane is only permeable to Na ions, Vm is the equilibrium potential for Na—ENa. Notice that ENa is a positive value since the ratio of [Na]o to [Na]i is a number greater than one so its logarithm is positive.

### 3. Record the values of ENa in different extracellular Na concentrations

As you did when you changed the [K]o, make a plot of ENa versus log [Na]o. In the Patch Parameters panel, change the extracellular [Na] from its default value of 140 mM to higher and lower values. Plot the value of the membrane potential versus the log [Na]o. Compare the slope of the line through the points you have plotted to the second figure shown in <u>this link</u>.

## WHAT DETERMINES THE "RESTING POTENTIAL" AND HOW DOES IT DEPEND ON ION CONCENTRATIONS?

A typical neuron is permeable to both K and Na ions, although far less so to Na than to K. What, then, determines the value of Vm at which the neuron "rests," Vrest?

(In this tutorial we have simplified the resting potential, whose value may be influenced by factors in addition to Na and K permeability. For example, the resting potential may have a contribution from "electrogenic" ion pumps that transport changes unequally across the membrane.)

### 1. Be sure that you have returned both the Na and K concentrations to their default values

Click the red box or checkmark associated with each concentration to return it to its default value.

### 2. In the P&G Manager, press the "Na and K Conductances" button

In the Patch Parameters panel, notice that the conductances, or channel densities, are now in the ratio of 1:1. Run the simulation. The resulting membrane potential, Vm, is the black line. Measure its <u>value</u> using the crosshairs option from the submenu. Why is Vm resting at this value?

### 3. Change the ratio of the conductances so that gK is greater than gNa

Set the K channel density, gK, to be 10, then 50 times greater than the Na channel density, gNa. Typically the ratio of gK to gNa at the resting potential can be about 50:1 in neurons. Notice that at this ratio, Vm rests near EK but is slightly depolarized to EK's value: gNa is making a contribution to the resting potential. If you could measure the Na and K *currents* flowing across the membrane at a gK:gNa ratio of 50:1, what would you <u>observe</u>?

### 4. Change the [K]o, keeping gK:gNa at 50:1

Change EK by changing the [K]o between 5 and 500 mM. Notice how Vm (= Vrest) tracks EK. From this experiment you can see how a change in serum [K] would affect the Vrest of cells. Because of the logarithmic relation in the Nernst equation, a change of 1 mM in the low values of [K]o have a much greater effect on Vm than a change of 1 mM at higher values. As you progress to the tutorials involving voltage-gated Na and K channels, you will see that the precise value of Vrest is absolutely crucial in determining what fraction of these channels are open, are closed and available for opening, or are closed and not available for opening.

### 5. Change the [Na]o

Return [K]o to its default value by clicking on the red mark. Divide the default value of [Na]o (140 mM) by two, then four or more, and re-run the simulation. <u>Why</u> is the resting potential so insensitive to the Na concentration?

## SIGNALS INVOLVE CHANGING CONDUCTANCE RATIOS

You can now imagine what will happen to Vm if you reverse the conductance ratio and make the membrane far more permeable to Na than K. In fact, by changing the value of the ratio with time, you can make any type of signal—from synaptic potential to action potential.

### 1. Make an "action potential"

Set the conductance ratio so that gK:gNa is 1:100. Now you should expect to see Vm come close to ENa. If you now reverse the ratio, such that gK:gNa is 100:1, Vm will return to very close to EK. This is the bare bones outline of what happens to make the action potential. In the <u>Na Action Potential</u> tutorial, you will study the clever mechanisms underlying how the changes in these conductance ratios enable the action potential to happen all by itself.

## NOW PRESS "QUIT" AND GO TO THE NEXT TUTORIAL

Press the "Quit" button in the P&G Manager.

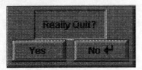

**REMEMBER!** *You must quit each simulation before going to the next one to avoid having multiple copies of NEURON running, each with a different simulation and set of panels, electrodes, and settings.*

# *The Na Action Potential*

## Target of Anesthetics and Toxins

### What is the "patch" action potential?

The action potential, or impulse, is a transient, regenerative voltage change—whether it propagates along an axon or simply happens in one location. The "patch" action potential is nonpropagating: It happens "in place," if you will. (Patch action potentials are sometimes called "membrane action potentials.") In subsequent tutorials in the "Axons" category, you will confront the complications of how the impulse travels.

### Depolarization triggers the action potential.

Injection of positive current by excitatory postsynaptic potentials (EPSPs) is the usual trigger of an action potential in neurons and muscle fibers. In this tutorial you will inject positive current into the patch with an electrode to trigger a Na action potential.

### A family of Na channel subtypes is now known to exist.

Hodgkin and Huxley discovered the Na conductance in the squid giant axon and described its properties. This Na channel, and the squid axon's K channel, are native, built-in channels in NEURON and are used throughout these tutorials. By the beginning of this century, nine subtypes of Na channel had been found in mammals. The Advanced Patch tutorial on Na and K Channel Kinetics displays their properties and allows you to explore how these properties affect membrane excitability.

### Goals of this Tutorial

- To observe the action potential and its underlying currents and conductance changes in a uniform patch of membrane
- To experiment with temperature, anesthetic agents, and toxins, and observe their effects on the action potential
- To examine the refractory period following the action potential and its consequences for membrane excitability

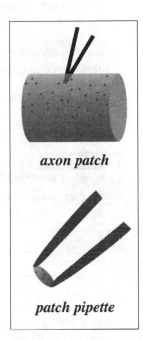

*axon patch*

*patch pipette*

# *Start the Simulation*

Click this button to bring up the panels and windows of the simulation.

**Start the Simulation**

# Description of the Panels and Windows Customized for this Tutorial

## 1. Assumptions

This tutorial assumes that you are now familiar with the following panels and manipulations:

- The function of the buttons within the P&G Manager and Run Control panels

- Running simulations by clicking Reset and Run (R&R) or clicking Reset and then the "Continue for (ms)" button in the Run Control panel

- Inserting a stimulating electrode by launching the Stimulus Control panel and controlling the onset, amplitude, and duration of the stimulus by selecting the "IClamp" option

**ATTENTION!** *If you close the Stimulus Control panel, you will remove the stimulating electrode from the patch. When you run a simulation, you will not observe an action potential in the Voltage-vs-Time graph but only a red horizontal line indicating the membrane potential. Reopen Stimulus Control to reinsert the electrode and stimulate the patch. Also, do not launch Stimulus Control more than once unless you intend to insert additional electrodes into the patch.*

- Storing, erasing, resizing, and measuring values on traces in plotting windows using the submenu features

- Using the field editor or the arrows box to change values in the Membrane Parameters panel

If this tutorial is your introduction to *Neurons in Action*, we suggest that you familiarize yourself with the panels and operations listed above by clicking their links.

## 2. Stimulus Control

A Stimulus Control panel is launched for you when you start the simulation; that is, a stimulating electrode is inserted into the patch. Select "IClamp" and notice the pulse parameters: The pulse is a "short sharp shock" with a duration of only 0.15 ms.

## 3. The Graphs

A Voltage-vs-Time graph is launched when you start the simulation. Other buttons in the P&G Manager will call up the other graphs as the tutorial progresses.

# Experiments and Observations

## GENERATE ACTION POTENTIALS

### 1. Press Reset & Run to generate an action potential

You will see an action potential displayed in the Voltage-vs-Time graph in black and two lines representing the equilibrium potentials for Na and K, ENa and EK, respectively. Remember that equilibrium potentials are calculated from the Nernst equation based on the external and internal concentrations of Na and K.

- The brief stimulating current pulse is shown in green.

- ENa is shown as a red line.

- EK is shown as a blue line.

## 2. *Observe the currents underlying the action potential*

Press Membrane Current Plots (in the P&G Manager) to bring up the appropriate graph and then run the simulation (press Reset & Run). You will see graphs of the Na and K currents (labeled "Patch INa" and "Patch IK," respectively) that flow during the rise and fall of the action potential.

If you are familiar with voltage clamp experiments, you will note that these action potential current patterns are not the same as those observed with a voltage clamp. The voltage clamp measures currents in response to the relatively simple stimulus of the voltage step (see Voltage Clamping a Patch tutorial); in contrast, the currents flowing during the voltage change of an action potential are more complicated.

## 3. *Now observe the conductances changing during the action potential*

Press Membrane Conductance Plots (in the P&G Manager) to bring up a graph for plotting the Na and K conductances ("Patch gNa" and "Patch gK") as a function of time. Run the simulation.

You could not make these observations of conductance with a current clamp or even with a voltage clamp in a real experiment. They may only be calculated.

## 4. *Question*

What underlies the depolarizing ramp at the beginning of the action potential?

## UNDERSTAND THE PECULIAR SHAPE OF INa

Why is INa so "kinky" with two phases? Why does it not have a smooth time course since the voltage and gNa—and even IK—all have smooth time courses? You can plot the driving force on Na ions to assist your reasoning.

## 1. *Plot the driving force on the Na ions (Vm minus ENa) as a function of time*

Press the "Plot Driving force for INa" button (in the P&G Manager). An appropriate graph will appear, overlying the Voltage-vs-Time graph. Run the simulation by pressing Reset & Run.

- The red line is ENa.

- The black line is the action potential.

- The brown line is the driving force on Na.

The driving force is large at Vrest (–120 mV) and decreases almost to zero during the action potential, then falls to an even greater value (–131 mV) during the undershoot of the action potential. Using the crosshairs option, click on the driving force trace and read off the time (the *x*-value) at which the minimum driving force occurs. (Read the value in the bar at the top of the graph.)

### 2. *Find the time at which the minimum (the notch) in INa occurs*

Clearly, INa begins to increase, then decreases to a minimum, and then increases again. Find the time at which this minimum occurs. Now find the *y*-value at that time on the action potential trace. Can you now explain the kink?

### 3. *Measure the size of the peak INa*

Are you perhaps surprised to find that the peak INa actually occurs on the falling phase of the action potential? Keep a note of this peak value for comparison with Na currents in the Voltage Clamping a Patch tutorial.

### 4. *Close the Plot-Driving-Force-for-INa graph*

Close this panel to expose the Voltage-vs-Time graph beneath it for the remainder of the experiments in this tutorial.

## MORE QUESTIONS:

### 1. *Would changing either the length or diameter of the patch alter the action potential in any respect? Should it?*

### 2. *Does the location of the stimulating electrode in the patch matter? Should it?*

### 3. *Suppose the membrane's capacitance were doubled*

Call up the Patch Parameters panel (in the P&G Manager) and change the value of the capacitance to see how your change would affect the shape of the action potential.

- When you change the capacitance, there will be changes in the rate of rise and in the final amplitude of the depolarization in response to the current pulse. Are these changes compatible with this explanation of capacitive currents?

- Restore the value of the capacitance to its default setting.

## STUDY THE EFFECT OF TEMPERATURE ON THE ACTION POTENTIAL AND UNDERLYING CONDUCTANCES

### 1. *Compare traces at different temperatures*

Use the "Keep Lines" option in all of the plots (right mouse-button submenu) for comparing traces. You must have your cursor positioned on the graph when you select "Keep Lines."

Note that your experiments so far have been carried out at 6.3°C, the standard reference temperature for squid—an invertebrate, used by Hodgkin and Huxley. Although the lack of heating in postwar (World War II) labs in England has been cited as a reason for this low temperature in their experiments, probably the most important reason was to slow the changes in the ionic currents to the point where the electronic circuits could control the potential more accurately.

**2. *Increase the temperature (in Run Control) by 10°C, then 20°C***

You can warm (or cool) the patch by using the "up" or "down" arrows (to the right of the white value field) or by typing a new value into the field using the field editor.

**3. *Draw conclusions from this important experiment***

What happens to the <u>duration</u> of the action potential if you change the temperature? Can you explain your observations by studying the effects of temperature on the underlying conductances? The results of this experiment are crucial for understanding why temperature affects the ability of an action potential to invade demyelinated regions of myelinated nerve (<u>Partial Demyelination</u> tutorial).

**4. *Return the temperature to its default value of 6.3°C***

## BATHE THE AXON IN ANESTHETIC AGENTS

**1. *Be sure that the <u>Patch Parameters</u> panel is open so that you can do more experiments***

Click on the "Patch Parameters" button (in the P&G Manager) if this panel is not already open.

**2. *Partially block both the Na and K conductances***

The anesthetics procaine and lidocaine reduce both the Na and K conductances by almost equal factors. Reduce the values of the conductances (Na channel density and K channel density) by a factor of two.

**3. *Compare the normal and partially blocked action potentials***

Using "Keep Lines," compare action potentials generated at different "concentrations" of anesthetic by continuing to divide by a factor of two. By how much must you reduce the two conductances to block the generation of the action potential? Make a note of this value for comparison with the experiments below using selective poisons of each channel type.

**4. *Return the Na and K conductances to their default values***

## BLOCK THE Na CHANNELS
## WITH THE POISON <u>TETRODOTOXIN (TTX)</u>

**1. *Block the Na channels***

TTX is a highly specific blocker of Na channels. Mimic the onset of its effects by gradually reducing the value of (only) the Na channel density. Divide repeatedly by a factor of two, as you did above, until the regenerative response disappears. Use "Keep Lines" to compare the action potentials in normal saline and at different degrees of block of the Na channels.

**2. *Question***

Which is more effective at blocking action potentials, a toxin that selectively blocks Na channels or the anesthetics (investigated above) that block both Na and K channels? <u>Why</u>?

**3. *Reset the Na channel density to its default value***

## HOW SOON CAN THE NEURON
## FIRE AGAIN AFTER AN ACTION POTENTIAL?

It is well known that there is a period of reduced excitability following an action potential, called the "refractory period." During this time, lingering changes in the ionic conductances following one impulse affect the threshold for firing the next impulse. The refractory period limits the frequency of impulses in a train of impulses.

### 1. Deliver two pulses to the patch: the first to evoke an impulse, and the second to test the duration of the refractory period

Set the Total # (ms) to 20. Then bring up a second "Stimulus Control" panel by clicking the button again in the P&G Manager. This action will put two electrodes into the patch—the simplest way for NEURON to inject two separately controlled current pulses. The second panel comes up below and offset from the first.

- Set the parameters for each pulse.

  - Delay: Deliver the first pulse at $t = 0$ ms and the second at $t = 9$ ms.

  - Duration: Keep each pulse at its very short duration (0.15 ms); this duration is approximately the same as that of transmitter-gated conductance changes that occur at fast synapses, explored further in the Neuromuscular Junction tutorial.

  - Amplitude: Initially keep both of the stimulus current amplitudes at 0.2 nA, above threshold for this duration pulse.

### 2. Measure how long the membrane is refractory

When you run the simulation, you should find that the second current pulse, occurring 9 ms after the first pulse, fails to generate a second spike even though the amplitudes of both stimuli are well-above threshold for setting up an action potential. Increase the delay of the second pulse until it generates an action potential. By doing this you should get a sense of how long the refractory period lasts.

### 3. Determine the degree of refractoriness at various times

Probe the refractoriness following the spike by decreasing the delay of the second stimulus to 9, 8, 6, 5, and 4 ms and finding the threshold current at each of these times.

You should find that you need more and more current to evoke the second action potential as you decrease the time between the two action potentials. No wonder an excitatory synaptic input has trouble generating an action potential when it falls into a refractory period!

### 4. Question

The responses to pulses at 6, 5, and 4 ms are particularly interesting. Can you explain the waveforms of the responses at each of these times?

# Threshold: To Fire or Not to Fire

## Treating Myasthenia Gravis

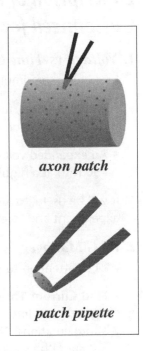

*axon patch*

*patch pipette*

### Why do we focus on threshold?

Threshold is a very important concept! Why should the neuroscientist have a clear understanding of threshold? First of all, it is key to brain function: Whether a postsynaptic potential is above or below threshold determines whether a neuron fires, and thus whether a muscle moves or a thought exists. Second, excitability abnormalities such as epilepsy have at their root a change in threshold. A thorough grasp of threshold is very important to understanding both pathological conditions and normal synaptic integration.

### Threshold and myasthenia gravis

In one particular pathological condition, myasthenia gravis, the neuromuscular junctions (NMJs) lose strength. Although the presynaptic action potential and the release of acetylcholine are normal, the number of postsynaptic receptors is abnormal. Thus, the acetylcholine is less effective at opening enough channels to bring the muscle fiber to threshold. One successful treatment for this disease prolongs the action of acetylcholine, making use of the relation between the threshold synaptic current and its duration. This tutorial will call attention to this relationship.

### Simulating threshold stimuli

An action potential may be initiated by depolarizing the cell's membrane in several ways: (1) The experimenter can depolarize the neuron or muscle fiber by injecting a pulse of current through an electrode, as we do in these simulations; (2) Excitatory neurotransmitter released from a presynaptic neuron can cause a conductance increase in a postsynaptic neuron or muscle fiber, giving rise to a postsynaptic ionic current; (3) Special channels in sensory receptors can depolarize the cell when activated; (4) Release from inhibition can depolarize the cell.

In this tutorial we will inject current via a synapse electrode to mimic postsynaptic events: brief postsynaptic potentials like that at the "NMJ," longer synaptic potentials due to transmitter-triggered intracellular cascades, the prolonged depolarizations of sensory receptor potentials, and finally, the "off responses" of neurons released from inhibition.

In textbooks it is often stated that an impulse will be generated whenever the membrane exceeds a certain fixed voltage level. Is this true? The experiments in this tutorial should enable you to draw a conclusion.

### Goals of this Tutorial

- To investigate whether threshold is at a fixed voltage in neurons
- To understand how threshold depends on the duration of the stimulus and the importance of this relation for synaptic transmission
- To explore the determinants of firing frequency in a train of action potentials generated by a sensory receptor potential

## Start the Simulation

Click this button to bring up the panels and windows of the simulation.

> **Start the Simulation**

## Description of the Panels and Windows Customized for this Tutorial

### 1. Voltage-vs-Time Graphs

Launching the simulation brings up two graphical windows:

- A conventional, full-scale plot displaying the voltage (from –70 mV to +50 mV) as a function of time

- An expanded voltage scale showing the threshold region (from –70 mV to –50 mV) at a higher resolution

It will be useful to Keep Lines in each of these graphs during a given experiment and to erase the stored traces between experiments.

### 2. P&G Manager

We call attention to three of the buttons in this panel:

- **Find Current Threshold:** Clicking this button will initiate a search algorithm to find the threshold current for a given pulse by successive approximations. The voltage finally displayed may be just subthreshold or just suprathreshold and will vary from search to search. This algorithm simply automates what you could do more painstakingly, and to more significant figures, by hand.

- **Plot Conductances:** Clicking this button will place a plot of the Na and K conductances below the Expanded-Voltage-vs-Time plot. Observing the ratio and timing of the conductances is crucial in understanding threshold.

- **Plot Currents:** Clicking this button will place a plot of the Na and K currents on top of the Expanded-Voltage-vs-Time plot. Observing the timing of the currents may also be useful in understanding threshold.

## Experiments and Observations

### IS THERE A CRITICAL CURRENT OR VOLTAGE THRESHOLD?

### 1. Give current pulses just below and above threshold

Before starting this experiment, select Keep Lines in both graphs. Depolarize your patch with current pulses just below and above threshold. (Notice that the pulse outlasts the 15 ms time of the x-axis because of its delay.)

- 2.4 nA (default setting)

- 2.486 nA (just below threshold)

- 2.500 nA (just above threshold)

- 2.600 nA (well above threshold)

## 2. Is there a critical stimulus current separating "all" from "none"?

It should be obvious that, indeed, there is a critical stimulus current threshold. But is there a critical voltage threshold?

## 3. Examine the traces in the Voltage-vs-Time graphs

- Are you able to find a critical value for the threshold voltage?

- Natural stimuli for neurons are currents that change the transmembrane voltage: synaptic currents, sensory receptor currents, or the currents surging down an axon in front of an action potential. In understanding whether a neuron will fire, one should think in terms of whether there is more or less current depolarizing the membrane rather than whether there is a voltage threshold.

## DOES THRESHOLD CHANGE WITH TEMPERATURE?

The default temperature for this tutorial is 6.3°C, the standard temperature for Hodgkin and Huxley's squid axon experiments. If you change the temperature, you would expect to change the kinetics of the opening, inactivation, and closing of the channels underlying the macroscopic currents and conductances. You might, then, expect to affect threshold: but in which direction will threshold change and by how much? Below, examine how threshold depends on temperature by looking at subthreshold and suprathreshold stimuli at two temperature extremes.

## 1. Find threshold for a very cold membrane patch

- Change the temperature in the Run Control panel to 2°C. Leave the pulse duration at 15 ms.

- Adjust the current until you find the values that elicit responses that are just subthreshold and just suprathreshold. NEURON will approximate these values automatically for you when you click the "Find Current Threshold" button in the P&G Manager. (You can do a more precise job yourself by successive approximations if you have the patience.)

- Write down the values of subthreshold and suprathreshold currents to compare with those at a higher temperature.

## 2. Find threshold at a higher temperature

- Repeat the experiment at 20°C, noting the current values that elicit sub- and suprathreshold responses.

## 3. Re-plot the two sets of traces, Keeping Lines, so that they may be compared

Clearly, threshold depends strongly on temperature. At the higher temperature, a several-fold increase in current is required to trigger the action potential; also, the rate of change of the voltage is steeper, and the action potential occurs much earlier in the pulse. Can you explain these observations?

This temperature experiment should have reinforced your observation that there is no fixed voltage threshold for an action potential.

The experiments in the next sections show how the stimulus required to bring a neuron or muscle fiber to threshold depends on the mode of excitation (whether excitation is brief or prolonged, and whether it is from a depolarizing synaptic potential or from release of inhibition) and the consequences for pathological situations.

Changes in temperature have a profound effect on impulse initiation and propagation and are clinically important, as you will see in the Partial Demyelination tutorial. An extensive discussion of the effect of temperature on the action potential is available.

*4. Restore the temperature to 6.3°C*

## TREATING MYASTHENIA GRAVIS

Stimuli for neurons range from brief (synaptic potentials lasting fractions of a millisecond) to long (synaptic potentials typically mediated by G-protein-coupled receptors) to sustained (receptor potentials of sensory receptors). For each of these potentials, what is the relationship between the duration of the stimulus and the amplitude of the underlying current that is needed to bring the membrane to threshold?

The NMJ offers an example where a large, brief synaptic current invariably brings the muscle fiber to threshold. But in myasthenia gravis, an abnormally low number of postsynaptic acetylcholine receptors leads to a decrease in the amplitude of this current. The treatment for this disease illustrates an important property of threshold: If you prolong the action of a neurotransmitter at a synapse, resulting in a postsynaptic current for a longer time, you actually need less postsynaptic current to bring the muscle fiber (or neuron) to threshold. We will explore this property below.

(Do not be concerned that the experiments here are performed at 6.3°C rather than at human body temperature: The principles are the same at either temperature.)

*1. Find the supra- and subthreshold currents for a very brief current pulse*

- **Set the pulse duration at 0.1 ms so as to mimic the brief end-plate current at the NMJ.**
  A depolarizing stimulus pulse of this duration is what neurophysiologists call a "short sharp shock." This duration is comparable to that of the acetylcholine-gated synaptic current at the NMJ, the "end-plate current" (EPC). You can experiment further with synaptic current in the Neuromuscular Junction tutorial.

- **Find the current required to bring the "muscle fiber" (the patch) to threshold for this short pulse.**
  Use your own successive approximations, or the "Find Current Threshold" button, to find the pulse amplitude that is just above threshold for generating an impulse. Compare this value to the default current value that brings the patch to threshold for the much longer pulse of 15 ms. Do you find this comparison surprising?

  ▪ Question: Why does the subthreshold voltage stay depolarized for such a long time before it finally returns to rest? The stimulus current lasts only 0.1 ms, yet the voltage change outlasts the stimulus duration by two orders of magnitude!

- Question: Will a few <u>neurotransmitter quanta</u> more or less make a difference in whether a synaptic potential near threshold causes a neuron to fire?

## 2. Mimic the treatment for myasthenia gravis

- This disease is treated by drugs that prolong the action of acetylcholine by blocking the enzyme that breaks it down—in other words, drugs that increase the duration of the synaptic current. This approach is quite effective since, as you can observe, if you double the duration of the stimulus you can halve the amount of current required to excite the cell.

- Increase pulse duration from 0.1 to 0.2 ms. By how much must you now <u>decrease the amplitude</u> of the current pulse (it was 84.5 nA at 0.1 ms) to bring a pulse of this duration to a subthreshold value?

## LONGER SYNAPTIC POTENTIALS

Synaptic potentials between neurons can last tens or hundreds of milliseconds if the receptor works through an intracellular signaling pathway or a transmitter lingers in the cleft. What important factors determine threshold for synaptic potentials in the range of tens of milliseconds?

## 1. Increase the stimulus duration to mimic slow synaptic currents

Observe threshold currents when the neuron is stimulated with long depolarizing pulses (tens of ms).

- **Lengthen the duration an order of magnitude.**
  Change the duration of the depolarizing current pulse to 1, 5, 10, and 20 ms and find the amplitude of the threshold stimulus for each duration by clicking the "Find Current Threshold" button. To accommodate the 20 ms pulse, you will need to change the time axis for this experiment by typing an appropriately larger number into the Total # (ms) field.

  - What <u>relationship</u> between duration and stimulus amplitude do you find in this time range? Is it different from that for brief pulses?

  - Why is the <u>shape of the subthreshold stimulus</u> the same for the 10 ms and the 20 ms pulse?

## MECHANOSENSORY RECEPTOR POTENTIALS

Mechanosensory neurons, such as those that detect touch, pressure, vibration, and pain, typically generate receptor currents of long duration while the stimulus is applied. The resulting long depolarizations set up trains of action potentials whose frequency typically encodes the strength of the stimulus. What factors influence this frequency?

## 1. Simulate the activity in a mechanoreceptor (e.g., a touch receptor)

Observe the onset of repetitive firing when the stimulus duration lasts for hundreds of milliseconds or seconds. Increase the Total # (ms) to 150.

- **Give a "brief touch" lasting 100 ms.**

  ▪ Increase the stimulus duration to 100 ms, a time that is very long compared to the duration of the action potential. Keep Lines and slowly increase the amplitude of the stimulus current. You should observe damped <u>oscillations</u> and then a train of impulses as the amplitude is increased.

- **Prolong the touch.**

  ▪ Find the lowest amplitude of the stimulus that evokes continuous firing throughout the pulse. Now increase the stimulus duration to 500 ms, a touch lasting half-a-second. Increase the Total # (ms) to 550. Again, slowly increase the amplitude of the stimulus current. Does the rate of firing encode the amplitude of the stimulus?

  ▪ (We are ignoring adaptation in our sensory neuron: The rate of firing is essentially uniform throughout the stimulus. In adaptation, the firing rate is high at the onset of the pulse and then decreases to a lower, steady value, involving additional types of channels.)

## HOW IS THE PEAK AMPLITUDE OF THE ACTION POTENTIAL AFFECTED BY NEARNESS TO THRESHOLD?

Action potential amplitude matters. There are certain processes that are drastically affected by small changes in spike amplitude. For example, small changes in the amplitude of the presynaptic action potential have been shown to have a large effect on the number of quanta released at the NMJ and, thus, on the postsynaptic response.

### 1. *Give a series of pulses of increasing amplitude*
Reset the stimulus parameters to their default values, where the current pulse is just below threshold and then, Keeping Lines, increase the amplitude of the stimulus in a series of steps so that the action potential is generated earlier and earlier in the pulse.

### 2. *Observe the values of the peaks*
Can you <u>explain</u> what happens to the peak of the action potential?

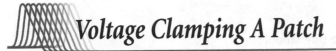

# Voltage Clamping A Patch

## Measuring Macroscopic Currents through Channel Populations

**The voltage clamp is the central tool of the neurophysiologist.**
The voltage clamp, conceived by Cole and used ingeniously by Hodgkin and Huxley, is a tool that has led to extraordinary advances in our understanding of the basis of electrical activity in nerve cells. It makes possible the study of currents through single ion channels.

**Hodgkin and Huxley's goal was to understand the mechanisms generating the action potential.**
They felt that they would understand the process if they could calculate an action potential from the experimental data they observed using the voltage clamp. With the voltage clamp, Hodgkin and Huxley stepped the voltage across the membrane to each of many voltage levels, held it there, and observed the currents flowing across the membrane at that voltage. At each voltage, a certain fraction of the population of Na and K channels opened and "macroscopic" currents flowed through those channels. From the observed currents, Hodgkin and Huxley developed the equations that allowed them to calculate the conductance changes underlying the action potential. We think every neuroscientist should know the history of their remarkable <u>experiments</u>, carried out in only three weeks but requiring analysis and calculations that took two years!

**NIA uses the equations derived from Hodgkin and Huxley's voltage clamp results.**
NEURON (and, thus, NIA) uses the Hodgkin-Huxley (HH) equations to calculate how the Na and K conductances change as a function of time for a given voltage step. It also calculates the currents, essentially reproducing the data that Hodgkin and Huxley observed.

## Goals of this Tutorial

- To plot currents in response to individual depolarizing voltage steps and to plot families of voltage steps.
- To plot the conductance increases (due to the opening, closing, and inactivation of the channels) in response to these voltage steps
- To experiment with "tail currents" (which give information on the time course of the closing of the channels when the voltage is returned to rest)
- To use the voltage clamp to demonstrate that a portion of the Na channels are inactivated at rest.
- To experiment with the effect of temperature on the kinetics of the conductance changes

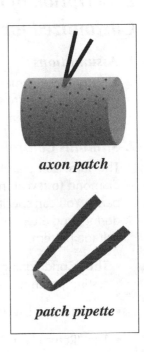

*axon patch*

*patch pipette*

# Start the Simulation

Click this button to bring up the panels and windows of the simulation.

**Start the Simulation**

# Description of the Panels and Windows Customized for this Tutorial

## 1. Assumptions

This tutorial assumes that you are now familiar with the panels and manipulations of *NIA*. Use the "Help with" pull-down menu on the side bar if puzzled at any point.

## 2. Stimulus Control: *The current-passing electrode*

The Stimulus Control panel comes up in the Location mode. Click the <u>VClamp</u> diamond to reveal the voltage clamp parameters in the bottom half of the panel. You can specify the amplitude and duration of the voltage before, during, and after the voltage step. The default settings specify the following voltage pattern:

- The "Conditioning Level" (holding potential) value equal to the usual resting potential, –65 mV

- The "Testing Level" (Command) value, a jump to 0 mV for 4 ms

- The "Return Level" value, –65 mV

## 3. Voltage-vs-Time graph: *The voltage clamp step*

The Membrane Voltage-vs-Time graphical window appears when you launch the simulation. Press R&R and you will see that the voltage is stepped from the "Conditioning Level" to the specified "Testing Level" and then returned. (If you instead see an action potential, IClamp is selected rather than VClamp in the Stimulus Control panel).

# Experiments and Observations

### OBSERVE THE Na AND K CURRENTS IN RESPONSE TO A STEP DEPOLARIZATION

## 1. Plot the currents in response to a voltage step to 0 mV

Bring up the Current-vs-Time plotting window by pressing Membrane Current Plots (in the P&G Manager). Run the simulation. You will observe the Na current (INa) and the K current (IK) as a function of time for the step from –65 mV to 0 mV and back.

## 2. Measure the peak Na current

Use the <u>Crosshairs</u> feature to make the measurements. How big is the Na current here? Keep Lines in order to compare this Na current with the peak Na current underlying the action potential in the next step.

### 3. Select IClamp and run the simulation to evoke an action potential and its underlying currents

The Na current during the action potential has two peaks, as you observed in the Na Action Potential tutorial. The larger of these peaks is only about 0.8 mA/cm$^2$, about half the magnitude of the peak current evoked by the voltage clamp step. What accounts for the difference in the magnitude of the Na current in these two situations?

### 4. Vary the Testing Level of the voltage pulse

Returning to VClamp, change the value of the depolarizing test pulse (using the VClamp menu in the Stimulus Control panel) in increments of, say, 10 mV. Find out how the peak INa varies with the level to which the voltage is clamped. Get out an old-fashioned piece of graph paper (or a graphing program like Excel) and plot the peak INa (y-axis) as a function of Vm (x-axis), then compare your plot with the classic figure from the work of Cole and Moore (1960).

## OBSERVE THE Na AND K CONDUCTANCE CHANGES IN RESPONSE TO A STEP DEPOLARIZATION

### 1. Bring up the Membrane Conductance Plots window

You can observe how the Na and K conductances change as a function of time during the step to 0 mV. Conductances must be calculated—they cannot be measured. NEURON calculates the conductance of each ion from the rate equations, and multiplies this conductance by the driving force on the ion to calculate its ionic current just as Hodgkin and Huxley did. Notice that this is simply Ohm's law.

### 2. Deliver the voltage step

Press R&R. The Na conductance (gNa) and the K conductance (gK) will be displayed on the same axis.

### 3. Explanations of the conductance kinetics are in the History section (see pulldown topics)

The kinetics of the conductances are not conventional. The description of the kinetics required the brilliance and insight of Hodgkin and Huxley. If you are eager to read about the kinetics at this point, you can pursue explanations of the sigmoid lag in the onset of each conductance and why there is no sigmoid lag when the membrane is repolarized to resting level.

## OBSERVE FAMILIES OF CURRENTS

### 1. Deliver 12 voltage steps from −40 mV to +80 mV

This experiment simulates a typical voltage clamp experiment (on a real neuron) in which preset protocols are run by computers. You will deliver a family of voltage steps and observe a family of currents. In the process of generating the display of these currents, NEURON will also calculate the underlying conductances.

- **Follow these steps to generate the family.**
  This family by default will be a series of 12 steps in increments of 10 mV starting from −40 mV (holding potential −65 mV).

- While still within the VClamp option (in the Stimulus Control window), set the Testing Level amplitude to –40 mV for the initial voltage level.

- Select VClamp Family. Notice that the "# of steps" button by default indicates 11, not 12. The first trace is the one for –40 mV and then there are 11 additional steps.

- Select the "Keep Lines" option in each of the plot windows.

- Press the "Vary Test Level" button, which is equivalent to pressing R&R.

- Re-size a plot with the View = plot option, if necessary.

**ATTENTION!** *You must press Vary Testing Level, not R&R, to generate a voltage clamp family. Run Control buttons apply only to individual runs.*

## 2. *Observe the time courses and amplitudes of the Na and K currents*

The Na currents at any level of depolarization precede the K currents. Where is threshold? You might want to read about the <u>first voltage clamp observations</u> where the lack of a threshold in the currents was originally pointed out.

The Na current family is rather complicated and will be sorted out by conducting further experiments below. The K currents are easier than the Na currents to observe as a family. Notice the changes in the time course and amplitude with greater depolarizations. Observe how the K currents relate to the K conductance changes: the conductances go through a maximum change and then approach saturation—that is, greater levels of depolarization cause only a negligible further increase in maximum conductance from the previous level. Yet the maximum currents continue to grow with level of depolarization. <u>Why</u>?

## 3. *Observe the Na currents by themselves*

To see the Na currents that may be under the K currents, you can delete the individual K traces by choosing the Delete option and clicking on the trace. Click Keep Lines again in each graph. Run the simulation. Clearly the inward Na currents grow to a maximum as the level of depolarization increases, then decline and eventually become outward although the conductance increases steadily to a maximum.

## 4. *Consider these questions about the Na current. Click <u>here</u> for answers*

- Why do the inward currents grow larger with depolarization, then smaller?

- What is special about the voltage at which the Na current is zero?

- Why are the currents outward at large depolarizations?

## 5. *Prepare for the next experiment*

Prepare for the next exercise by closing and reopening all the graphs for plotting currents and conductances so that the ability to plot K currents is restored. Return the Testing Level pulse amplitude to its default value of 0 mV.

## OBSERVE "TAIL" CURRENTS

What is a tail current and what is its importance? Do the following series of experiments to find out.

### 1. Observe Na and K tail currents

Observe currents and conductances at the offset of a voltage step to 0 mV (upon its return from the Testing Level to the Return Level).

- **Follow these steps to generate a big tail current:**

  - Select VClamp in the Stimulus Control window.

  - Be sure the Testing Level pulse amplitude is at its default value of 0 mV.

  - Reduce the duration of the Testing Level pulse to 1 ms. (Leave the Conditioning Level pulse at 0.5 ms and the Return Level pulse at 100 ms.)

  - Select Keep Lines in each graph to preserve these traces for the next experiment.

  - Press R&R (you are delivering a single pulse, not a family).

- **Make your observations and try to figure out what causes a tail current.** Observe the direction, amplitude, and time course of the currents, especially the Na current, at the end of the pulse. (You may have to use View = plot.) In addition to being at the tail end of the pulse, the Na current at this time point really looks like a tail! Increase the time resolution by setting the Total # ms to 2. Comparing the time course of decay of the Na tail current with that of gNa should give you a big hint as to what causes the tail current.

### 2. Get more information: Determine how the tail currents depend on voltage

Clamp to three different Return Levels (for example –20 mV, 0 mV, and +20 mV) to see how the magnitudes of the currents depend on the voltage level. Again, the behavior of the Na and the K currents is very different. Can you now formulate an hypothesis to account for your observations and explain tail <u>currents</u> (before checking the link!)?

### 3. Consider these questions:

- <u>What causes the Na tail current to jump</u> to a value that is larger than the value just before the the end of the pulse?

- Can the amplitudes of the jumps in Na tail currents be used to <u>measure the time course of gNa during the step</u>? Remember that gNa cannot be measured directly; it may only be calculated. This is done by dividing the current at any time point by the driving force.

## DEMONSTRATE INACTIVATION OF THE Na CONDUCTANCE

### 1. How does inactivation of the Na channels depend on voltage?

At the normal resting potential of –65 mV, about 40% of the HH Na channels are inactivated. Hyperpolarization removes inactivation with time;

at a much greater resting potential (for instance, –100 mV), none of the channels will be in the inactivated state. On the other hand, a depolarized holding (conditioning) potential will shift more of the channels to the inactivated state.

Note: The voltage level preceding a test pulse is standardly referred to as the "conditioning level" as it is here. When the duration of this pulse becomes long enough so that the channels are in a steady state (about 3 ms at 6.3°C for the HH channels), the conditioning pulse may be referred to as the "holding potential."

## 2. Set pulse parameters for observing inactivation

You can observe the consequences of inactivation by generating a family in which the Conditioning Level is changed but the Testing Level is kept constant. Adjust the parameters of the clamp step as follows:

- Select VClamp and set the Conditioning Level amplitude to –100 mV.

- Set the Test Level amplitude to 0 mV.

- Select VClamp Family from the Stimulus Control window.

- Set the # of steps to 11 (remember, there will actually be 12 traces).

- Set the # mV/step to 5.

- Make certain Keep Lines is selected for all of the graphs.

## 3. Generate the family by pressing Vary Conditioning Level

A family of Na currents and a family of K currents will be plotted. You can expand the time axis by increasing the Total # (ms) to 2.

## 4. Look carefully at the Na and K conductances and currents

Should the current <u>patterns</u> during the pulse mirror the conductance patterns for each ion?

## OBSERVE THE EFFECT OF TEMPERATURE ON THE Na AND K CONDUCTANCE KINETICS

Cooling the preparation will cause the channels to open and close more slowly and, conversely, warming it will speed up the kinetics of the conductances.

## 1. Restore default settings

Return all pulse parameters in VClamp and VClamp Family to their default settings. Erase the graphs but continue to Keep Lines. Leave the Total # (ms) at 2. Run the simulation to deliver a pulse from –65 mV to 0 mV and back, as at the beginning of this tutorial.

## 2. Increase the temperature in increments of 10°C

Increase the temperature by 10° to 16.3°C, then 20°C, and re-run the simulation at each temperature. Observe how the change in temperature affects the kinetics of the conductances and therefore the currents.

Hodgkin and Huxley found a three-fold change in the <u>rate constants</u> underlying both the Na and the K conductances (and currents as well) for each 10°C change. This important observation is at the heart of the interpretation of all of the experiments in the *NIA* tutorials in which you change the temperature.

## LEARN ABOUT THE LIMITATIONS OF THE VOLTAGE CLAMP

At this point you might want to read the section on <u>limitations</u> of the voltage clamp technique, caused by the "series resistance" through which the current must flow. In this linked section, <u>ideal</u>, <u>typical</u>, and <u>out-of-control</u> clamps are illustrated and discussed. In addition, the tutorial on on <u>Voltage Clamping Cells</u> allows you to experiment with series resistance in the electrode and within an intact cell (rather than a patch).

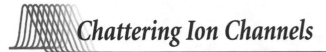

# Chattering Ion Channels

Patching Single Na and K Channels

**One could argue that the basis of life lies in ion channels.**
With the help of ionic pumps that establish the transmembrane voltage, ion channels control so many of the processes fundamental to a living organism. Perhaps using transporter proteins a different sort of life could be established, but it would be so slow!

**This tutorial will enable you to experiment with single channels.**
You can study the behavior of single Hodgkin-Huxley (HH) Na and K channels, which are the voltage-gated ion channels that underlie the action potential in squid axons and most other axon types. These channels are only two of the many different subtypes of Na and K channels currently described, but certainly two of the very crucial ones. The understanding of single-channel behavior gained in this tutorial should permit you to readily identify variations employed by other channels, giving rise to a diversity of functions.

**Here, you will simulate patch clamp experiments.**
Until Neher and Sakmann invented the patch clamp technique in 1976, we could only imagine how these postulated channels might open and close. Did they open like a circular valve, a small hole expanding gradually into a larger one? Did they open in a series of transitions? Was there a molecular stopper that plugged and unplugged the channel? Using the patch clamp, it was fantastic to see the square-shaped currents that showed the channels flipping in an instant between an open and closed state. Perhaps this tutorial can convey some of the excitement of seeing channels in action and finding out how they behave.

**Goals of this Tutorial**
- To observe, measure, and understand the features of the currents flowing through single, voltage-gated Na and K channels
- To appreciate the stochastic nature of the gating of single channels by voltage
- To understand, through experimentation, how depolarization favors the open state of the channel
- To conceptualize how macroscopic currents, in populations of many channels, arise from the aggregate behavior of the microscopic currents through individual Na and K channels

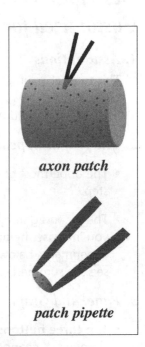

*axon patch*

*patch pipette*

## Start the Simulation

Click this button to bring up the panels and windows of the simulation.

**Start the Simulation**

## Description of the Panels and Windows Customized for this Tutorial

### 1. Assumptions

This tutorial assumes that you are now familiar with the basic manipulations of the panels and graphs and that you know how to Keep Lines, Erase, use the Crosshairs, and use View = plot within the graphs.

### 2. The graphs appearing upon launching the simulator

- The uppermost graph, Voltage vs Time, simply displays the voltage-clamp step.

- The second graph displays the Single Channel Currents vs Time. When you increase the number of a given type of channel beyond 3 or 4 in the experiments below, you will have to use View = plot in the submenu to see the summed currents.

### 3. Panel and Graph Manager

- **Top three buttons:** You can record from a patch containing either Na channels, K channels, or both channel types (default). Each button calls up a Current-vs-Time graph displaying <u>single channel currents</u> from a patch containing that particular channel type.

- **Normalized current plot:** This button calls up a graph in which the current is normalized so that the summed currents may be viewed when you have many channels in the patch. Plots of the macroscopic Na and K currents are continually displayed in this graph so that the summed single-channel currents may be compared to them.

- **Extend time axis:** With this button you can call up a Current-vs-Time graph in which a long pulse (110 ms default) is delivered to the patch, permitting you to observe many single-channel openings.

### 4. Stimulus Control

Using a <u>single electrode clamp</u>, this voltage clamp panel controls the duration and value of the three levels of the voltage clamp: the Conditioning Level, the Testing Level, and the Return Level.

### 5. Patch Parameters

In this panel you control the number of Na and K channels in the patch as well as the Na and K conductances and equilibrium potentials. When you specify one channel type by its button in the Panel and Graph Manager, the conductance of the other channel type will automatically be set to zero.

**PLEASE NOTE!** *In order to "remove" a channel from the patch, set its conductance to zero, not its number; setting its number to zero will give you meaningless results.*

# Experiments and Observations

### OBSERVE SINGLE Na AND K CHANNELS IN A PATCH

By default, you start with a patch containing a single Na channel and a single K channel.

## 1. Record both Na and K currents in response to a depolarizing voltage step

- **You have isolated a patch.**
  With considerable skill, you have successfully isolated an <u>outside-out</u> patch of membrane where you hope to observe single Na and K channels. Your external bathing solution has typical extracellular Na and K concentrations and the solution inside the pipette has typical intracellular concentrations, establishing the values of ENa and EK shown in the Patch Parameters panel. Your recording situation is arranged so that currents that would flow inward are negative-going.

- **Voltage clamp your patch.**
  Holding your breath, you press R&R to <u>clamp</u> the patch from –65 mV to –11 mV (a value halfway between ENa and EK). Do you observe single channel currents (middle graph)? If you don't, press it again...and again: Channel openings are probabilistic. Are there two types of current in the patch that might correlate with what you have <u>learned</u> about Na and K currents in the <u>Na Action Potential</u> tutorial?

## 2. Study the opening and closing of these channels

- **Observe the form of the channel openings.**
  Does each channel open and close slowly so that the conductance gradually increases and then decreases? Does it open in steps? Or does it snap open and then maintain a certain value of conductance until it closes? Until the patch clamp, we really didn't know. Imagine the thrill Neher and Sakmann must have felt upon seeing these "square" openings for the first time in 1976. The blips on the rising and falling phases of the voltage step and channel currents are due to the computer plotting algorithm.

- **When does each channel type open?**
  If you press R&R repeatedly, you should observe that the time until opening for each channel is unpredictable. So, then, does the depolarizing step "<u>open the channel</u>"?

- **What if you do not apply a depolarizing voltage-clamp step?**
  You can test what happens without a depolarizing voltage-clamp step by setting the Testing Level to –65 mV, the same value as the resting potential and the Conditioning Level. Now, press R&R repeatedly to see if any channels are opening without depolarization. Do you observe channel openings? <u>Should you</u>?

## STUDY A SINGLE K CHANNEL BY ITSELF

### 1. Press "K channel only" in P&G Manager

This is equivalent to putting tetrodotoxin in your external saline to block the Na channels in the patch. In the Patch Parameters menu, note that the gNa is now set to zero.

- **Voltage clamp your patch.**
  In the Patch Parameters Panel, notice that there is one channel in the "# K channels" field. Depolarize the patch from –65 mV to –11 mV in Stimulus Control, then press R&R. Keep pressing R&R until you see channel openings. What is the evidence that you are observing a K channel (other than the writing on the button)?

- **Are there two current amplitudes?**
  If your channel opens toward the end of the pulse, you might observe two amplitudes of current, and your first thought might be that there are two conductance states for this K channel. But look closely: Does the smaller current actually occur after the voltage step is turned off? Might it be that both currents are occurring during the same prolonged channel opening, an opening that is outlasting the voltage step? If you don't understand what is happening, the experiments below should help.

- **First, focus only on the channel openings that close before the depolarizing step ends.**
  Change the value of the step depolarization. We suggest stepping to –40 mV, –20 mV, 0 mV, and +20 mV. (Expand the current axis with View = plot on the graph submenu to make your events larger, if you wish.) Be sure you understand three key observations of these single-channel currents as you increase the amplitude of the depolarizing step.

### 2. What determines the amplitude of the current flowing through the K channel when it opens?

- **Prepare to measure the current as a function of voltage.**
  When you do this you will discover, experimentally, that channel currents obey Ohm's law.

  - **Measure the current flowing through the open channel at each voltage.** (Click on the current trace and observe the $y$-axis value in the top bar of the graph.)

  - **Record the value of the current and the voltage step (on paper).** Remember that you are only examining the current through a single K channel—your Na channel is blocked with tetrodotoxin. Does the K current through the channel become larger or smaller as the step voltage moves farther away from the value of EK (EK = –77 mV: see Patch Parameters panel)?

  - **Plot your values of current versus the voltage step values.** Current should be on the $y$-axis, and voltage should be on the $x$-axis. Are your values in a straight line? If they are, why is the line straight? Extrapolate the line to see where it crosses the voltage axis (current = 0). What is the significance of the voltage value at this crossing point?

- So, did the current get bigger as the voltage moved away from EK or moved closer to EK? As you clamp to a voltage closer to EK, the "driving force" on the K ion (Vm – EK) will decrease. You can play with this concept by changing the value of EK as well in the Parameters Menu.

- **Questions:**

  - Do you understand why you observe a smaller amplitude of current at the offset of the pulse if the channel opening outlasts the pulse?

  - What should you observe if you step the voltage to a value negative to EK?

  - Will the single channel conductance change with voltage?

  - Is conductance a value you determine by measurement or by calculation?

## 3. Observe the effect of membrane potential on the time that the channel spends in the open state

Compare the durations of channel openings at –25 mV and at +40 mV during a very long test pulse.

- **Press the "Extend Time Axis" button to bring up a graph that extends the *x*-axis (to 120 ms, by default).**
  Pressing this button will also automatically change the duration of the test voltage clamp pulse to 110 ms. Note that the Total # (ms) (in Run Control) is now 120 ms.

- **Run the simulation with your test pulse at –25 mV.**
  The channel will open and close repeatedly. The durations of the channel's open states probably appear random. Indeed, they are; if you were to patiently measure the durations of a large number of events, put them in duration bins, and plot the number of events in each bin versus event duration, you would find that the shortest durations occurred with the highest frequency and that the distribution fell off exponentially, as is characteristic of a plot of stochastic events.

- **Save a trace using Keep Lines. Run the simulation again with the test pulse at +40 mV.**
  Because the driving force at the two test potentials is different, the amplitudes of the currents will be different, and you should be able to easily distinguish the durations of the openings at each potential. Observe any difference in the open times of the channel at the two potentials and explain your observations.

  If you were now to measure the durations of a number of these events and again plot the number of events in each duration bin versus event duration, you would find a new exponential distribution at this new membrane potential. This type of measurement of open (and also closed) durations has enabled the modeling of the number of states (conformational changes in the protein) through which a channel passes as it opens and closes, the forward and backward rate constants between states, and their dependence on membrane potential.

- **Close the Extended Time Axis graph and reset all default settings.**

## STUDY A SINGLE Na CHANNEL BY ITSELF

### 1. Press "Na channel only" in the P&G Manager

This is equivalent to putting TEA (tetraethylammonium ion) in your external saline to block the K channels in the patch. In the Patch Parameters menu, note that gK is now set to zero.

- **Study one channel (specified by "1" in the "# Na channels" field of the Patch Parameters panel).**
  Depolarize the patch from –65 mV to –11 mV in Stimulus Control, then press R&R. Keep pressing R&R until you see channel openings.

  - When, during the pulse, does the Na channel tend to open?

  - How does this time, at which the Na channel tends to open, compare to that of the K channel?

  - How does the average open time of the Na channel compare to that of the K channel? Explain any difference.

  - Are there Na channel openings late in the pulse? If there are very few, why is this?

  - When a channel closes, can you <u>tell whether it has truly closed</u> or whether it has become inactivated?

  - Summarize the <u>evidence</u> that you are observing a Na channel (rather than a K channel), and think of other experiments you could do to glean more evidence.

- **As you did above for the K channel, explore how the current through the Na channel depends on voltage.**

  - Change the value of the step depolarization to –40 mV, –20 mV, 0 mV, +20 mV, +40 mV, and +60 mV.

  - Plot your values of current versus the voltage step values. Are they in a straight line? Does it cross the voltage axis? What voltage value is this crossing point?

## INCREASE THE NUMBER OF CHANNELS IN THE PATCH

### 1. Press "Both Na and K channels" in the P&G Manager

- **Observe two channels of each type.**
  Enter "2" in the "# Na channels" and "# K channels" fields of the Patch Parameters panel.

- **Depolarize the patch from –65 mV to –11 mV in Stimulus Control.**
  Press R&R repeatedly. Sometimes you will see only one Na or K channel opening. Sometimes, however, you will see the two single-channel currents adding together, indicating that the two channels have both opened at nearly the same time. If you observe two channel openings but they are separated in time and do not sum, can you tell whether one channel opened twice or both channels opened?

- **Observe how recruiting single channels builds up the macroscopic currents.**
  Call up the "Normalized current plot" graph (if you have not already done so) to observe how adding more and more "chattering channels" to the patch gives rise to the macroscopic Na and K currents plotted in the graph. Add a third channel of each type and give successive pulses to observe the openings.

- **Increase the number of each channel type to 10.**
  Make sure you understand:

  - Why the ensemble of channel openings looks so different from trial to trial

  - Why there tend to be more openings of K channels later in the pulse

  - Why all of the Na channel openings seem clustered at the beginning of the pulse, with openings at the end very rare

## 2. *Increase the number of channels in the patch to the hundreds, then thousands*

- **Go for it: Increase the number of channels to 100 each and then 1000 and then 10,000.**
  You should see how the macroscopic currents, observed in the Patch Voltage Clamp Tutorial, emerge as the "ensemble average" of the opening of these many channels. While any one channel behaves stochastically, the opening of the population of channels yields an ever-smoother current plot as the number of channels is increased.

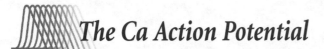

# The Ca Action Potential

## How to Make a Long, Cardiac-like Action Potential

**Voltage-gated Ca channels can support action potentials.**
Since the 1950s we have known that certain cell types can generate Ca-dependent action potentials. Voltage-gated Ca channels, rather than Na channels, underlie the regenerative rising phase of some action potentials and prolong the falling phase of others. The driving force on Ca is enormous because of its extraordinarily low concentration inside the cell. Consequently, opening Ca channels can result in a huge inward Ca current.

**Ca channels comprise many subtypes.**
Many subtypes of voltage-gated Ca channels have now been identified, revealed by molecular biology and patch clamping. A lucid summary of the identity and properties of these channels and their families as of 2001 can be found in Hille (2001). In this tutorial you will use a commonly found channel, the high-voltage-activated L-type Ca channel from the CA3 pyramidal neuron of the hippocampus (Migliore et al. 1995). This channel has been imported into *NIA* from the ModelDB (modeling database) of the NEURON website.

**Cardiac action potentials depend on the properties of Ca channels.**
Ca entry during action potentials, through a variety of Ca channel subtypes, is used to trigger or regulate various cell functions. Examples include the secretion of hormones and neurotransmitters, muscle contraction, and pacemaking. In this tutorial, you will experiment with prolonged action potentials to simulate those in cardiac muscle. Although the action potentials in cardiac pacemakers and in ventricular myocytes are extraordinarily complex, involving many different ion channels and pumps, and cannot be simulated here with precision, it is possible to gain an understanding of how the presence of Ca channels in these cells gives rise to the long and unusual cardiac action potentials.

**Goals of this Tutorial**
- To generate a Ca-dependent action potential and observe its special characteristics, particularly how it differs from a Na-dependent action potential
- To generate a hybrid action potential and observe the contributions of the voltage-gated Na and Ca channels to its various phases
- To mimic the basic features of the cardiac action potential

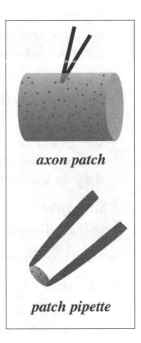

*axon patch*

*patch pipette*

## Start the Simulation

Click this button to bring up the panels and windows of the simulation.

> **Start the Simulation**

## Description of the Panels and Windows Customized for this Tutorial

### 1. Assumptions

This tutorial assumes that you have done the Na Action Potential tutorial.

### 2. The Panel and Graph Manager

- **Top three buttons:** These buttons allow you to choose whether your patch contains Na channels only (default), Ca channels only, or both channel types (each at one-half normal density).

- **Cardiac-like AP:** Clicking this button sets the ratio of the Na/Ca conductance to approximate the prolonged duration of an action potential in cardiac ventricular myocytes.

- **Sum of Currents Plot:** Clicking this button brings up a graph in which the sum of the currents through the K channels and the Na or Ca channels is plotted as a black line.

### 3. The graphs

Launching the simulation brings up two graphical windows:

- A Voltage-vs-Time plot

- A Currents-vs-Time plot where the Na, Ca, and K currents may be plotted

Later in the tutorial you will be asked to call up the "Sum of Currents" plot, which will appear beneath the other two graphs.

### 4. Stimulus Control

Call up the parameters of the current pulse (click IClamp), and note that the default pulse is a "short sharp shock" with a delay of 0.1 ms, a duration of 0.1 ms, and an amplitude of 0.2 nA.

### 5. Patch Parameters panel

In this panel you can change: (1) the capacitance, (2) the default Na, Ca, and K channel densities (conductances) and the leak conductance, and (3) ENa, EK, and Eleak.

## Experiments and Observations

### COMPARE Na-DEPENDENT AND Ca-DEPENDENT ACTION POTENTIALS AND THEIR UNDERLYING CURRENTS

In this experiment you will first record a Na-dependent action potential (default) in a patch containing only Na channels. Then you will switch to a patch containing only Ca channels and evoke a Ca-dependent action potential.

### 1. Press R&R to record a Na-dependent action potential and its underlying currents

Note in the Patch Parameters panel that the default Ca channel density, or Ca conductance (gCa), is set at zero. Click Keep Lines in each of the graphs so that you may next compare the Ca action potential and its underlying currents with those of the Na action potential.

### 2. In the P&G Manager, press Ca channels only

In the Patch Parameters panel, the gNa is now set to 0 S/cm$^2$ and the gCa is given a value.

### 3. Press R&R to try to elicit a Ca-dependent action potential

If you keep the same stimulus parameters as those that elicited the Na action potential, you will observe the voltage response is subthreshold. What is a <u>possible explanation</u> for this failure?

### 4. Increase the current amplitude in order to bring the patch to threshold

Increase the current amplitude in steps of 0.1 nA until you see changes in the falling phase of the Ca action potential. What is <u>happening</u>? Continue to increase the current amplitude in steps of 0.1 nA until your action potential no longer changes shape. By examining the underlying currents, you should be able to understand how they <u>shape the action potential</u>.

### 5. Look at a plot of the sum of the Ca and K currents

Press the "Sum of Currents Plot" button in the P&G Manager to bring up a new graph in which the summed currents are plotted as a black line. This plot should make it obvious why the action potential finally returns to rest after its long plateau: A slight imbalance in the two currents, due to their different kinetics, leads to a surge in the K current which allows it to <u>win the battle</u> resoundingly and shut down the depolarization emphatically!

### 6. Compare the Na and Ca action potentials

- Set the stimulus current amplitude to 1.0 nA—a large current, which will depolarize the patch to +30 mV. This large depolarization will open all Na channels when the "Na Channels Only" button is pressed, or all of the Ca channels when the "Ca Channels Only" button is pressed.

- Choose "Na Channels Only" and press R&R to elicit a Na action potential and its currents. Remember to Keep Lines.

- Now choose "Ca Channels Only," and elicit a Ca action potential with its currents.

- What are the main <u>differences</u> between the Na and Ca action potentials and their currents?

### 7. Generate a Ca action potential by increasing the duration of the default stimulus instead of its amplitude

- Return the amplitude of the current pulse to its default value of 0.2 nA.

- Increase the duration of the pulse in steps of 0.1 ms.

- <u>Compare</u> the Ca action potential generated by increasing the duration of the stimulus with that generated by increasing its amplitude (above).

### 8. Restore the duration of the stimulus to its default value

## EXPERIMENT WITH HYBRID ACTION POTENTIALS
## IN WHICH BOTH Na AND Ca CARRY THE INWARD CURRENT

From the experiments above comparing Na and Ca action potentials, you can appreciate that a mixture of these channel types would lead to a "designer" action potential specialized for the function of a particular neuron. How fast do you want the action potential to rise, for example? Increase the Na channel density to speed it up or the Ca channel density to slow it down. Should it be longer (relatively more Ca channels) or shorter (relatively more Na channels)? In this section, design your action potential by varying the Na and Ca conductances.

1. *Press the "Na and Ca Channels" button in the P&G Manager, then press R&R to observe a hybrid action potential*

   The depolarization lingers at threshold long after the 0.1 ms stimulus is over, then finally takes off, peaks at +28.4 mV, declines slowly for about 1.5 ms, then the patch repolarizes rapidly. For this default action potential, the Na and Ca conductances have each been set at half their normal density.

2. *Observe how the underlying currents shape the action potential*

   From your observations above, and from those in the Na Action Potential tutorial, you should be able to answer these questions:

   • Why does the Na current (INa) (red trace) have two phases?

   • The dip in the INa occurs at $t$ = 1.4 ms. What is the action potential doing at this moment?

   • Why is the Ca current (ICa) (brown trace) so delayed?

   • Why does the ICa turn off faster than the INa even though Ca channels do not inactivate and Na channels do?

3. *Change the Ca channel density (gCa), keeping the Na channel density (gNa) constant*

   We suggest you start with 0.01 S/cm$^2$ and increase gCa in steps of 0.01 or 0.02. Can you answer the following questions?

   • Are you changing the percentage of channels that are open in the population, the density of open channels, or both?

   • As you increase gCa, what happens to the plateau of the action potential, and why?

   • Are you affecting the rising phase of the action potential? Why or why not?

4. *Change the value of gNa, keeping gCa constant*

   First make moderate changes. Start with 0.01 S/cm$^2$ and increase gNa in steps of 0.01 or 0.02.

   • What is the most obvious change in the action potential as you increase gNa?

   • Does increasing gNa affect the repolarization of the action potential, and, if not, why not?

### 5. Increase gNa again, this time in a higher range

Start with 0.2 S/cm$^2$ and increase gNa in steps of 0.2 (still keeping gCa constant).

- The membrane now depolarizes very quickly into the range in which the Ca channels open (–30 mV and above). Does this mean that the ICa now contributes to depolarizing the patch?

- The time course of repolarization of the membrane now seems to vary with gNa. Why is this?

- Click here if you are unsure about the answers to all of these questions about changing gNa.

## SIMULATE THE CARDIAC ACTION POTENTIAL

There are two basic types of cardiac action potential: the action potential of the pacemaker system and that of the muscle fibers (myocytes) of the ventricle. Here, we simulate the prolonged action potential of the myocytes, where the initial depolarization is due to Na channels and the plateau to both K channels and L-type Ca channels. (Other channels and pumps make the real cardiac action potential more complicated, but these three currents give the action potential its fundamental features.)

### 1. Press the "Cardiac-like AP" button

This action will set the Na and Ca channel densities at a reasonable ratio for the cardiac action potential. If you now press R&R, you will find that the action potential is longer than the 5 ms time base. Increase the "Total # (ms)" while you re-run the simulation until you see the action potential repolarize.

### 2. Observe the current amplitudes and time courses

Use View = plot to rescale the currents. Notice how small the INa is compared with the ICa and IK. In heart muscle, the inward ICa triggers further release of Ca from intracellular stores, which then causes contraction.

### 3. Examine the sum of the currents

You should observe a small surge of outward current at the beginning and end of the action potential but otherwise a remarkably perfect balance between the inward ICa and the outward IK.

# The Neuromuscular Junction

## The Classic Model of Synaptic Excitation

**This tutorial simulates the responses of a muscle fiber to acetylcholine (ACh) released from the motoneuron's presynaptic terminal.**
The simulations model the postsynaptic (or "end plate") membrane of the well-known neuromuscular junction (NMJ) of the frog. At the NMJ, ACh binds to its postsynaptic (nicotinic) receptors, which are also ion channels. The channels open, causing a postsynaptic "end plate current" (EPC) to flow that leads to a postsynaptic, depolarizing "end plate potential" (EPP) in the muscle fiber.

**ACh-gated receptors are permeable to both Na and K ions.**
Activation of ACh receptors causes a simultaneous and equal increase in the postsynaptic conductance to both Na and K ions. In this tutorial you will see the relationships between the ACh-gated conductance, the resulting EPC, and the EPP.

**Studying the NMJ reveals general principles of excitatory synapses.**
In later tutorials you will experiment with excitatory postsynaptic potentials (EPSPs) in neurons, such as: the interaction of EPSPs In a patch, the spread of an EPSP along a dendrite to the soma and axon, and the temporal integration of more than one EPSP.

**Goals of this Tutorial**
- To observe the relationships between the ACh-gated conductance, the resulting current (the EPC), and the voltage change in the muscle fiber (the EPP)
- To experiment with the reversal potential of the ACh-gated EPC and EPP
- To discover the effect on the EPP of adding voltage-gated channels to the muscle fiber

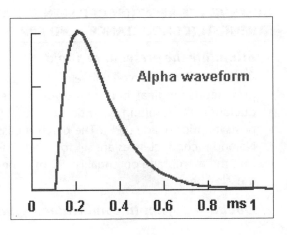

*patch with synaptic input*

## Start the Simulation

Click this button to bring up the panels and windows of the simulation.

**Start the Simulation**

## Description of the Panels and Windows Customized for this Tutorial

### 1. NEURON's representation of a postsynaptic potential

The conductance change caused by ACh has the kinetic form shown to the right. Since this form is often

Alpha waveform

| 0 | 0.2 | 0.4 | 0.6 | 0.8 ms 1 |

represented mathematically by a function called the alpha function, in NEURON it is referred to as the AlphaSynapse.

The AlphaSynapse panel controls the parameters of the synaptic input as follows:

- **onset:** the time of onset of the synaptic potential in ms

- **Tpeak:** the time to peak of the synaptic conductance change in ms

- **gmax:** the maximum synaptic conductance in µS

- **e:** the reversal potential, set by default at −15 mV for the ACh-gated channels

## 2. The graphs

A Postsynaptic Conductance-vs-Time graph shows the conductance change caused by the ACh.

- A Postsynaptic Current-vs-Time graph plots the postsynaptic currents through the ACh-gated channels.

- A Postsynaptic-Voltage-vs-Time graph plots the membrane potential, Vm. Its time course and amplitude will depend on:

  - The time course and amplitude of the current

  - The capacitance and resistance of the postsynaptic membrane

## 3. The Patch Parameters panel

Notice that the tutorial begins with the Na and K channel densities set to zero and only a leak conductance in the membrane.

## 4. Stimulus Control

When launched during the tutorial, this panel "inserts" a stimulating electrode and controls a current pulse delivered to the postsynaptic membrane patch. When this panel is launched, there are then two ways of injecting current into the patch: (1) through the postsynaptic ACh-gated channels, controlled by the AlphaSynapse panel, and (2) through the electrode, controlled by the Stimulus Control panel.

# Experiments and Observations

## OBSERVE THE RELATION BETWEEN SYNAPTIC STRENGTH (CONDUCTANCE) AND EPP AMPLITUDE

### 1. Stimulate the presynaptic input

When you click R&R you will release a small amount of ACh from a virtual presynaptic terminal; in response you will see a change in the synaptic conductance, the resulting synaptic current (EPC), and a small change in the postsynaptic voltage (EPP). The patch is passive; the Hodgkin-Huxley (HH) Na and K conductances are set to zero by default. (Notice in the Reset field that the membrane potential is −90 mV, the typical resting potential of a muscle fiber.)

### 2. Double the synaptic conductance (gmax) several times

Double the conductance, choose Keep Lines in each plotting window, and re-run the simulation. Keep doubling the conductance up to 64 μS (or above). You will see that there is no further significant increase in the amplitude of the voltage even though the synaptic conductance and current continue to increase.

When John ("Jack") Eccles, Bernard Katz, and Steve Kuffler observed the EPP in frog muscle fibers in 1941, they had to include curare in the bathing medium to reduce the EPP's amplitude below threshold for eliciting an action potential in the muscle. You need not worry about using curare because the HH channels in your patch have zero conductance for now.

### 3. *Explain the results of this experiment*

- The time courses of the synaptic currents can have considerably shorter durations and different shapes than those of the conductance changes. Why?

- The time course of the voltage change, the EPP, is much slower than either that of the synaptic conductance change or of the synaptic current. Its peak is reached when the current returns to zero! What shapes the time course of the EPP?

- Clearly, as the conductance increases, the EPP approaches an asymptotic value. What is the significance of this value?

### 4. *Compare your observations with a figure from a classic paper*

If you re-run your simulation with Total # (ms) set to 30, you can compare your voltage changes to the uppermost trace in Figure 5 of the classic study of the EPP by Paul Fatt and Bernard Katz in 1951. In their case, the muscle is curarized and the EPP is subthreshold. Consult this link for a simulation of how an EPP would spread along the muscle fiber, as in the Fatt and Katz experiments.

### 5. *Return gmax to its default value of 2 μS. Erase the traces from your previous experiment*

## DETERMINE THE REVERSAL POTENTIAL OF THE ACH-GATED EPP

### 1. *Time the EPP to arrive during a pulse of injected current*

To observe reversal of the EPP you will have to change Vm to different values with a prolonged current pulse. The EPP can then be timed to occur after the pulse has reached a steady state.

- **Set the Total # (ms) to 25.**

- **Insert a current-passing electrode into the patch.**
  Bring up the Stimulus Control panel. Check the pulse parameters in IClamp. The duration of your depolarizing current pulse has been set at 25 ms (that is, it terminates just off the graph) and its amplitude initially is set at 5 nA.

- **Time the EPP.**
  In the AlphaSynapse panel, change the onset of the EPP to 20 ms so that it will occur after the depolarized voltage response has reached a steady state.

### 2. Run the experiment

Using Keep Lines in all of the plotting windows, deliver a set of depolarizing current pulses to the patch, increasing the amplitude of the current pulse with each R&R in 5 nA steps to 50 nA from its initial value of 5 nA. What is the value of the reversal potential?

- **Use View = plot to expand the conductance and current trace amplitudes.**
  The amplitudes of the conductance and current traces will be small. Expand them and examine them. What determines the amplitude of each current?

- **Expand the time base of a selected region.**
  You can expand the region around the reversal potential on any graph by choosing New View on the pop-up menu (right mouse button). Use the left mouse button to box the interesting area. Resize the box; pull it out horizontally to see the events on a faster time base, or vertically for more *y*-axis resolution.

## HOW DO VOLTAGE-SENSITIVE CHANNELS AFFECT THE SHAPE OF AN EPP OR AN EPSP?

The next experiments will use a patch containing HH Na and K channels rather than a passive patch. In the muscle fiber, depolarization of the postsynaptic end-plate region must gate the Na and K channels in the surrounding membrane to elicit an action potential and cause contraction.

### 1. Set the Total # (ms) to 10 and reset the default parameters

You may have to bring up new windows to replace those in which you employed View = plot. The Patch Parameters panel should be open.

### 2. Click the "Add HH channels" button (in the P&G manager)

Clicking this button will reset three parameters as follows:

- The densities of the Na and K channels will be changed to the standard HH values.

- The stimulus current will be set to zero.

- The synaptic conductance (gmax) will be changed to 3.532 µS, just below the threshold level of 3.533 µS for generating an impulse.

### 3. Run the simulation

Click R&R to see the waveform of an EPP in an active patch membrane. If you "increase the number of transmitter quanta" by increasing gmax the slightest bit, to 3.533 µS, this EPP will (after prolonged deliberation) generate an action potential.

A very small difference in the transmitter-gated current can determine whether or not the postsynaptic membrane fires. You may remember this result from the Threshold tutorial. Remember, also, that at threshold the Na and K currents can be equal and opposite for quite some time, as you see here, before one of them gains the advantage. Note that many milliseconds passed between the increase in ACh-gated conductance (and the resulting increase in current) and the postsynaptic action potential it triggered.

### 4. Question

Can you explain the shape of your subthreshold EPP in this active membrane? If you are puzzled about EPP or EPSP shapes observed experimentally when recording from intact muscle fibers or neurons (rather than a patch), a detailed explanation is available in this link.

### 5. Compare EPPs in a passive and active patch

If you wish to compare this EPP in an active patch (containing the voltage-gated Na and K channels) with that in a passive patch, bring up the Parameters Panel to reset the conductances of the Na and K channels to zero.

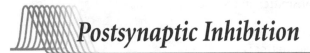

# Postsynaptic Inhibition

## The GABAergic Synapse: Target of Psychoactive Drugs

**Inhibitory postsynaptic potentials (IPSPs) in the CNS are primarily due to the neurotransmitter GABA (gamma aminobutyric acid).**
Many mental disorders are thought to be due to disturbances in postsynaptic inhibition. Seizures, anxiety, and depression, for example, are treated with drugs that enhance or interfere with the action of GABA. Even alcohol affects GABAergic transmission. It is crucial for the neuroscientist to understand how postsynaptic inhibition works.

**GABA and other inhibitory transmitters "clamp" a cell's membrane potential at a value below the threshold of the action potential.**
IPSPs do not simply subtract from EPSPs, they make a cell less excitable. GABA and other inhibitory transmitters cause a conductance increase to either Cl or K, depending on the receptor, tending to clamp the cell at ECl or EK. In this tutorial you will experiment with inhibition to see how IPSPs dampen excitability in this manner. In later tutorials you can experiment with the interaction of IPSPs and EPSPs <u>in a patch</u> or in the <u>dendritic arbor</u> of a cell.

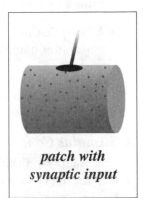

*patch with synaptic input*

**Goals of this Tutorial**
- To understand how an IPSP "clamps" the membrane voltage
- To understand disinhibition
- To probe what happens to membrane excitability following an IPSP

# Start the Simulation

Click this button to bring up the panels and windows of the simulation.

> **Start the Simulation**

# Description of the Panels and Windows Customized for this Tutorial

### 1. The synaptic input

The graphs and panels of this tutorial are similar to those of the <u>Neuromuscular Junction</u> tutorial except that the resting potential, (in the "Reset" field of the Run Control panel), is set to –65 mV, as is characteristic of neurons, rather than to –90 mV, typical of muscle fibers.

The <u>AlphaSynapse</u> panel controls the parameters of the IPSP as follows:

- **onset:** the time of onset of the IPSP, in ms

- **Tpeak:** the time to peak of the synaptic conductance change, in ms

- **gmax:** the conductance change caused by the inhibitory transmitter, in µS

- **e:** the reversal potential for the current through the transmitter-gated channels. The default reversal potential for the inhibitory transmitter is –65 mV.

## 2. *The graphs*

- A Synaptic Conductance-vs-Time window shows the conductance change caused by inhibitory transmitter.

- A Synaptic Current-vs-Time window plots the currents through the transmitter-gated channels.

- A Voltage-vs-Time window shows Vm. Notice that the voltage scale extends from –80 mV to +20 mV since the resting potential is –65 mV, the value for the squid axon and a typical value for neurons.

## 3. *Stimulus Control*

Upon launching this panel, you will have two ways of injecting current into the patch: (1) through the postsynaptic GABA-gated channels, controlled by the AlphaSynapse panel, and (2) through the stimulating electrode "inserted" in the postsynaptic membrane patch and controlled by the Stimulus Control panel.

# *Experiments and Observations*

### OBSERVE THE CONDUCTANCE, CURRENT, AND VOLTAGE CHANGE (IPSP) IN RESPONSE TO A PULSE OF INHIBITORY TRANSMITTER

An IPSP typically results from an increase in conductance to K or Cl ion. Thus, the IPSP has a reversal potential ("e" in the AlphaSynapse menu) at ECl or at EK and the IPSP's reversal potential is either at, or negative to, the resting potential. Even though there is a conductance change due to the action of transmitter, there may be no voltage change if Vm is exactly at the reversal potential for the IPSP. (Yet it is still called an IPSP.)

## 1. *Deliver a pulse of GABA by clicking R&R*

When delivering your pulse, you can think of it as GABA released from a presynaptic, inhibitory neuron or as GABA spritzed from a micropipette onto the postsynaptic membrane. You should see the conductance change caused by the GABA, but do you also see a synaptic current or a change in voltage (an IPSP)?

## 2. *Increase the "amount" of GABA delivered by increasing gmax (µS) in the AlphaSynapse menu*

Double the conductance from 2 to 4 µS; double it again, then again. Your conductance should increase, but do you see a synaptic current or an IPSP? Although there is an increase in conductance, both Vm and e are at –65 mV. Thus there is no driving force, no current, and no voltage change.

This conductance increase, however, would be expected to make coincident depolarizing inputs less effective. This topic is explored in the Postsynaptic Interactions tutorial.

## REVEAL THE IPSP

An experimenter may miss observing such inhibitory inputs onto a cell. The wise investigator, however, will displace the membrane potential away from its resting value to test for the presence of these hidden events. Put yourself in this position.

### 1. Insert a stimulating electrode by launching Stimulus Control

Checking IClamp, you will see that it will deliver a depolarizing pulse 25 ms in duration with an amplitude of 5 nA. This pulse will displace the voltage away from the reversal potential of the IPSP.

- Change the time scale on the graphs so that you can see this pulse: Set the Total # (ms) in the Run Control panel to 30.

- Set the onset of the IPSP in the AlphaSynapse panel so that it occurs during the plateau of the depolarization (15 ms is good).

- Now run the simulation. The IPSP, occurring during the plateau of the current pulse, should be obvious.

### 2. Reverse the IPSP

Next, deliver a hyperpolarizing current pulse by changing the amplitude of the stimulating pulse to −5 nA. You should see a reversed IPSP. (Remember that View = plot will allow you to view hyperpolarizing pulses that may have gone off the bottom of the graph.)

## EXCITE A CELL BY DISINHIBITING IT

There are many synapses in the CNS where action potentials are evoked when a neuron is released from inhibition. This phenomenon is called "disinhibition" and the action potential (or burst of action potentials) generated is sometimes referred to as an "off response."

### 1. Click the "Add HH Channels" button in the P&G Manager

A new Postsynaptic Voltage-vs-Time plot will appear on top of the previous graph and the standard Na and K channel densities will be set in the Patch Parameters panel, converting the patch from passive to active membrane. In the AlphaSynapse menu, gmax ($\mu$S) will be set automatically to zero so there is no synaptic input for this experiment.

### 2. Mimic prolonged inhibition

Inhibition is often prolonged, caused by trains of IPSPs or continuously released GABA. Mimic this inhibition by injecting a hyperpolarizing current pulse (instead of using the AlphaSynapse menu).

- Set the pulse duration to 10 ms and the amplitude to −3 nA.

- Gradually increase the hyperpolarizing current (to −4, −5, etc.), Keeping Lines, until something interesting happens.

- Do you agree with the authors' <u>observations and explanations</u> in this experiment?

### 3. Compare the off-response impulse with one generated by a depolarizing pulse

Store off-response traces generated just below and just above threshold. Then generate a similar set of traces using a depolarizing pulse (current settings of 3.3 and 3.4 nA will work for this 10 ms pulse). <u>What is different</u> about the action potential (threshold, amplitude) in these two cases and why?

## ARE THERE CHANGES IN EXCITABILITY FOLLOWING AN IPSP?

If inhibition lasts long enough, it can lead to the removal of inactivation from voltage-gated Na channels, which leads to a post-stimulus hypersensitivity to excitation. Just after the inhibitory period, there is a brief window of time for a depolarizing synaptic potential to have a greater effect on the neuron. This subject is explored in greater depth in the <u>Interaction of Synaptic Potentials</u> tutorial. In the present tutorial you can begin to experiment with this phenomenon.

### 1. Insert a second electrode into the patch (bring up a second Stimulus Control panel and displace it from the first)

You can generate inhibition with the first electrode and test excitability with the second electrode.

- In the first Stimulus Control panel (mimicking the IPSP), set the pulse duration to 10 ms and the amplitude to –4 nA. This pulse will mimic a prolonged IPSP but only cause a subthreshold off-response.

- In the second Stimulus Control Panel (evoking a test action potential), set the duration of the stimulus to 0.1 ms, and the amplitude of this "short sharp shock" to 100 nA. This pulse will evoke a just-suprathreshold impulse in the absence of a preceding IPSP.

- Set the Total # (ms) to 50 so you can test the excitability of the membrane over this long time.

### 2. Map the membrane excitability following the hyperpolarizing pulse

Use the second pulse to test the excitability of the membrane following the hyperpolarizing pulse. Set the delay of the second pulse to 18 ms and then increase the delay by 4 ms until 42 ms (don't stop before 42 ms). Can you <u>explain</u> these rather complex results?

# *Interactions of Synaptic Potentials*

## Na Channel Kinetics Complicate Synaptic Interactions

### How do synaptic potentials interact?

Can an excitatory postsynaptic potential (EPSP) or an inhibitory postsynaptic potential (IPSP) influence the subsequent excitability of a neuron? In this tutorial you will investigate how these synaptic potentials can have an impact on whether or not a subsequent EPSP causes a neuron to fire.

### This tutorial focuses on "temporal summation," the interaction of EPSPs and IPSPs in time.

These experiments explore the interaction of synaptic potentials that essentially interact at the same point. Two EPSPs might come from two spatially close presynaptic inputs or from two sequential action potentials in the same neuron. An EPSP and an IPSP would naturally come from an excitatory and an inhibitory input located close to one another on the cell. Tutorials in the "Cells" section of the "Advanced" tutorials address interactions in space as well as time.

### Synaptic interactions can be complicated by time-dependent conductance changes.

Excitatory and inhibitory neurotransmitters typically cause conductance changes that are straightforward. But the resulting voltage changes open, close, or inactivate voltage-gated channels in the postsynaptic membrane that then affect the actions of subsequent synaptic potentials. In this tutorial you can look at the underlying currents and conductances to understand what might otherwise be puzzling changes in voltage during synaptic potential interactions.

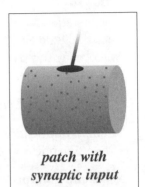

*patch with synaptic input*

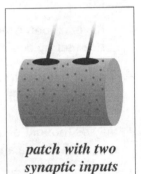

*patch with two synaptic inputs*

### Goals of this Tutorial
- To observe how EPSPs sum in a passive membrane
- To experiment with summation of EPSPs in an active soma membrane (membrane containing voltage-gated Na and K channels)
- To discover how both EPSPs and IPSPs can affect subsequent membrane excitability
- To realize that EPSPs can be inhibitory and IPSPs can be excitatory, contrary to accepted nomenclature

## *Start the Simulation*

Click this button to bring up the panels and windows of the simulation.

**Start the Simulation**

# Description of the Panels and Windows Customized for this Tutorial

## 1. Assumptions

This tutorial assumes that you have completed the experiments in the Threshold, Neuromuscular Junction, and Postsynaptic Inhibition tutorials.

## 2. The graphs

The Voltage-vs-Time graph is initially set up for a passive patch. When you click the "Add HH Channels" button in the P&G Manager, a similar graph will overlay this passive-membrane window, but this new graph is set up for active membrane. A Conductance-vs-Time graph is also available.

## 3. The two AlphaSynapse panels

- **The synaptic inputs:** The two AlphaSynapse panels, [1] and [2], represent two synaptic events in the patch.

- **Default conductances:** The default conductance setting for EPSPs is 0.5035 µS. This value is just below threshold for generating an action potential in active membrane at 6.3°C.

- **Reversal potential:** The reversal potential for EPSPs in this tutorial has been set by default to zero for simplicity.

## 4. The Patch Parameters panel

A Patch Parameters panel allows you to change channel densities (conductances) and ion concentrations. The postsynaptic membrane patch may be thought of as an isopotential soma. Notice that this tutorial begins with both the Na and the K conductances set to zero, as appropriate for a passive membrane.

# Experiments and Observations

## SUMMATION OF EPSPS IN A PASSIVE POSTSYNAPTIC MEMBRANE

### 1. Deliver two EPSPs to the passive patch

How do two EPSPs, caused by two sequential action potentials in the presynaptic neuron, interact when the postsynaptic membrane is passive? Clearly there is no presynaptic neuron in this simulation; instead of shocking the presynaptic nerve, you will specify the times of arrival, or onsets, of the postsynaptic conductance changes.

### 2. Run the simulation with the default settings

The onset of the first EPSP occurs at 0.5 ms and that of the second at 10 ms, after the first has decayed.

### 3. Decrease the time between the EPSPs

Gradually reduce the time of onset of the second EPSP, AlphaSynapse[2], from 10 ms to 0.5 ms. Remember to Keep Lines. Is summation linear? That is, is the peak amplitude of the simultaneous EPSPs at 0.5 ms double that of one EPSP?

### 4. Double the conductance of each EPSP

See if your observations hold for greater conductance changes. Double, then triple the conductance for both EPSPs. Since the membrane is passive, <u>will summation always be linear</u> for any conductance change?

### 5. Restore default settings to prepare for the next experiment

## SUMMATION OF EPSPS IN A POSTSYNAPTIC MEMBRANE WITH VOLTAGE-GATED Na AND K CHANNELS: TIME IS OF THE ESSENCE!

### 1. Add the Na and K channels

Clicking the "Add HH channels" button will add the Na and K conductances automatically and also set the value of gmax for the second EPSP (0.555) to a value about 10% above threshold. The first EPSP remains at 0.5035 μS, slightly below the threshold value.

### 2. Open the Conductance-vs-Time and Expanded Conductances windows

Looking at the conductances should be useful as you consider explanations of your observations. These two graphs plot the conductances at two different gains. Both are needed since there is an order of magnitude difference in the amplitudes of the conductance changes occurring during the synaptic potential and during the action potential.

### 3. Deliver the two EPSPs

Since the first EPSP is just below threshold, the depolarization lingers near threshold for some time before the K current wins over the Na current and the patch repolarizes. You should not be surprised by this long time of decision if you have completed the <u>Threshold</u> tutorial. But what about the response to the second EPSP? Why does this EPSP not generate an action potential? Look at the conductances to answer this question.

(You can assure yourself that the conductance setting for this second EPSP is truly above threshold by setting the gmax of the first synaptic input to zero and running the simulation. Remember to restore its default value afterwards.)

### 4. Delay the second EPSP

Over what period of time does the first EPSP affect the ability of the second EPSP to generate an impulse? Generate a family of traces by delaying the second EPSP by, say, 2 ms intervals, and look at the underlying conductances. Remember to Keep Lines.

### 5. Consider mechanism and terminology

There are two matters to think about in this experiment. The first is to ask <u>what mechanisms</u> can explain your observations. But the second has to do with how our terminology in neurophysiology may restrict our thinking. Wasn't the first EPSP actually *inhibitory* in this experiment? Perhaps a more accurate name for EPSPs would be "DPSPs," "depolarizing" rather than "excitatory" postsynaptic potentials. Since we seem to be stuck with the EPSP terminology, we hope this tutorial has at least broadened your expectations of what an EPSP can do to the neuron.

## COMBINING TWO SUBTHRESHOLD EPSPS

When two just-subthreshold EPSPs occur synchronously, clearly the result will be an EPSP that generates an action potential. But what happens when the second event is delayed with respect to the first?

### 1. Start with simultaneous EPSPs at 1 ms. Leave the HH conductances turned on

Set the onset times of both EPSPs to 1 ms and restore each of their conductances to the default subthreshold value (0.5035 µS). Plan to record the conductances at high and low gain for each run. Using Keep Lines is especially valuable in this experiment.

### 2. Increase the temporal separation of the EPSPs

Generate a family by increasing the time of onset of the second EPSP by 2 ms for each run until the action potential fails. In the low-gain Conductance-vs-Time graph (the middle graph) you see the full amplitudes of the the Na and K conductances. Looking at this graph, and at the high-gain "Expanded Conductances" graph, <u>explain</u> the changes in the amplitudes of the action potential and the conductances that you observe.

### 3. Further increase the EPSP separation

Now increase the time of onset of the second EPSP further, until at least 17 ms. First, what do you predict will happen? Are you surprised by what actually happens and can you <u>explain</u> it? Change the Total # (ms) to 35 and keep increasing the separation of the EPSPs. As you watch what is happening, remember that these are two *subthreshold* EPSPs. To explain what you observe, measure the K conductance with the crosshairs at rest and at 17 ms and look carefully at the voltage at the interesting timepoints.

## WHAT ARE THE EFFECTS OF AN IPSP ON MEMBRANE EXCITABILITY?

An *inhibitory* postsynaptic potential can also affect a subsequent EPSP. It is common to find inhibitory and excitatory synapses side by side on a neuron, essentially at the same location electrically. Converting the first synapse to an IPSP here, you can experiment with its effects on a subsequent EPSP.

### 1. Make the first synapse inhibitory

Set its onset time to the default value of 0.5 ms and set its reversal potential, e, to –80 mV. You can leave its conductance unchanged at first, but experimenting with the conductance would also be instructive.

### 2. Make the second event a subthreshold EPSP

Time it to occur at 10 ms, substantially after the IPSP. Confirm that it is subthreshold, if you wish, by setting the conductance of AlphaSynapse [1] to zero.

### 3. Deliver the IPSP and the EPSP

Can you <u>explain</u> your observation? Hint: Before you consult the link, change the reversal potential of the IPSP and observe what these changes do to the EPSP. If the reversal potential is at the resting potential of –65 mV, for example, what is the consequence for the EPSP?

## VOLTAGE-DEPENDENT CONDUCTANCES CAN
## INTRODUCE COMPLICATIONS INTO SYNAPTIC INTERACTIONS

Your experiments should have revealed at the very least an inconsistency in the nomenclature of synaptic designations!

Activation of synapses whose reversal potentials are more positive than the resting level cause depolarizing currents to be injected into a cell, whereas synapses whose reversal potentials are more negative than the resting level cause hyperpolarizing currents to be injected. Depolarizing currents are in the direction of eliciting a spike and have accordingly been designated as "excitatory"; hyperpolarizing currents have been designated "inhibitory."

You have seen, however, that for a period following its peak, a depolarizing current can actually suppress the response of the cell to subsequent supra-threshold EPSPs under certain conditions. Conversely, an IPSP can be followed by a period of increased excitability. Nonlinear conductances are responsible.

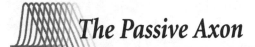

# The Passive Axon

## How Voltages Spread in Axons without Voltage-Sensitive Channels

**How far do voltages spread without an action potential?**

From the experiments in this tutorial on the passive decay of a voltage along an axon illustrated in the diagram below, you will be able to appreciate the necessity for a mechanism to enhance the voltage spread. Nature discovered voltage-sensitive ion channels and with them was able not only to enhance voltage spread but to generate a signal, the action potential, whose shape and amplitude are maintained with high integrity. This integrity will be clear in the next tutorial on propagation in a uniform unmyelinated axon (Unmyelinated Axon Tutorial).

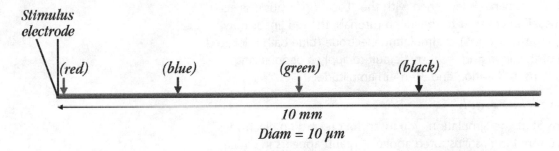

**Are there types of neurons in which voltages spread only passively, without action potentials?**

Yes. Two examples in the human body are the rod and cone photoreceptors of the retina, and hair cells—the sensory receptors of the inner ear. These sensory cells are so short that action potentials are not needed to get signals from one end to the other.

**Goals of this Tutorial**

• To observe the passive spread of a voltage change along an axon in response to injected current
• To measure the "length constant" of the axon
• To experiment with how membrane resistance and axon diameter affect the passive spread of a voltage
• To investigate whether a change in membrane capacitance affects passive spread
• To observe passive spread when the electrode is located at different positions along this "closed-ends" axon

## *Start the Simulation*

Click this button to bring up the panels and windows of the simulation.

> **Start the Simulation**

## *Description of the Panels and Windows Customized for this Tutorial*

### 1. *Assumptions*

This tutorial assumes that by completing the Basic Patch tutorials you are familiar with the *NIA* panels and manipulations. The Passive Axon tutorial is the first of the tutorials in the Axons section that allow you to run movies of the spread of voltages and propagation of the action potential along squid and frog axons.

### 2. *Stimulus Control*

The Stimulus Control panel is launched with the "Location" option selected by default, as usual. In contrast to the Patch tutorials, the red line is now long, representing the axon. The stimulating electrode (blue ball) is located at the left end of the axon and is set by default to apply a depolarizing current pulse 20 ms in duration and 30 nA in amplitude.

### 3. *The Voltage-vs-Time graph*

When you press Start the Simulation, you insert four recording electrodes into an axon 10 mm long as illustrated above. A graph appears in which voltage will be plotted versus time at these four locations along the axon. The four recording electrodes are color-coded to their traces as follows, with numbers in parentheses indicating their relative distance from the left end:

- red: (0)

- blue: (0.25)

- green: (0.5)

- black: (0.75)

For simplicity, in this case of a passive axon, depolarizations are shown as changes from a resting level of zero.

## *Experiments and Observations*

### AT FOUR LOCATIONS ALONG THE AXON, OBSERVE VOLTAGE RESPONSES TO THE CURRENT PULSE

### 1. *Depolarize the axon at its left end*

Press R&R and use the slider to select the speed at which you wish to run this simulation. You will observe the voltage recordings at the four electrodes. How does the rate of rise and the amplitude of the voltage step <u>change</u> as you record it farther and farther away from the point of stimulation?

(Note that the voltage change at the recording electrode at the [0.75] position [three-quarters of the way down the axon from the point of stimulation] is too small to be observed at this gain.)

### 2. *Increase the gain and re-run the simulation*

To increase the gain on the voltage axis, press the "V vs Time, Expanded" button. This action brings up another graph with an expanded voltage axis.

When you run the simulation again, you can note more accurately the time of onset of the voltage change as it spreads down the axon. You may be surprised to find that a voltage spreading passively has a delay associated with the attenuation of the voltage signal.

## OBSERVE A MOVIE OF THE VOLTAGE CHANGE AS IT SPREADS ALONG THE AXON

### 1. *Call up the Voltage-vs-Space graph*

A unique feature of the *NIA* tutorials is their ability to show voltages spreading or propagating in the neuron. As you prepare to watch the "movie" on this new graph, remember that the *x*-axis is now distance, not time.

### 2. *Press R&R to run the movie*

Here you can appreciate the spread of a voltage change along the passive axon and relate these changes in space to the voltages recorded (as a function of time) at each electrode.

## MEASURE THE LENGTH CONSTANT (*L*) OF THE AXON

### 1. *What is the <u>length constant</u>?*

The length constant *L* is not a physical property of the membrane; it is arbitrarily defined as the distance over which the voltage decays to approximately one-third of its initial value, or, more precisely, to 1/e (0.368) of its initial value:

$V = (Vo) * (exp[-x/L])$

To measure it you will have to freeze the voltage decaying over distance (in the next step).

### 2. *Capture a trace from which you can measure the length constant*

Do this by stopping the movie when the voltage at the left end (red trace in the Voltage-vs-Time plot) has reached a steady-state (maximum) level while the stimulus is still on. You will then be able to observe that the voltage in the Voltage-vs-Space plot falls off exponentially. A simple way to do this is to set the "Total # (ms)" button to 19; this will stop the simulation just before the end of the 20 ms stimulus pulse.

### 3. *Make your measurements*

- Using the crosshairs, measure the *x* and *y* values on the Voltage-vs-Space graph.

- Measure the initial value of the voltage at *x* = 0.

- Move the crosshairs to the voltage at 1/e (0.36788) of this initial value. The spatial resolution chosen for this simulation may not allow you to reach your calculated number precisely. Nevertheless, the value of *L*, which you read nearest to this value, is accurate to within 1%.

**CAUTION!** *The term "length constant" is useful for describing voltage spread in passive processes. But it applies ONLY to membranes that are linear resistances—axons without voltage-sensitive channels, or that are operating in a range where voltage-sensitive channels are not open. When voltage-sensitive channels are active, the current-voltage relation of the membrane is nonlinear and the "length constant" equation and name lose their meaning.*

## HOW DOES THE LENGTH CONSTANT CHANGE WITH MEMBRANE RESISTANCE?

### 1. *Bring up the Axon Parameters panel*

The length constant depends on the ratio of the membrane resistance to the axial resistance (resistance of the axoplasm). You can change the membrane's passive resistance by changing leakage conductance in this panel to determine how such changes affect passive decay.

### 2. *Decrease the membrane resistance*

Decrease the membrane resistance by, say, a factor of four by multiplying its leakage conductance by this factor. Your intuition probably tells you that if the resistance is lower, current will not spread as far down the axon. But how quickly will it decline? It is instructive to actually see this experiment as a movie!

### 3. *Run the simulation*

What are the new values of the initial voltage, the voltage at 1/e of the initial voltage, and the length constant? How does this value of length constant compare with your original measurement?

If you want instead to *increase* the membrane resistance, the higher membrane resistance will drive your current pulse off scale. Check the link for instructions.

### 4. *Reset the leakage conductance to its default value*

Click on the red box next to the "Leakage cond." button.

## HOW DOES THE LENGTH CONSTANT CHANGE WITH AXON DIAMETER?

### 1. *Change the axial (internal) resistance by changing the diameter*

The axial resistance depends on the specific resistance, or resistivity, of the axoplasm and the diameter of the axon. Again, intuition should tell you that the larger the diameter of the axon, the more easily current will flow along it, and thus the lower the axial resistance will be. Here, you can experiment with changes in diameter to get a feeling for how the voltage spread depends on diameter.

- **Increase the diameter fourfold to 40 μm.**
  Remember that axons of larger diameter require more current to depolarize them to the same value as that recorded in an axon of smaller diameter (next step).

- **Increase the amplitude of the stimulus current.**
  We suggest an eightfold increase to restore the voltage response to approximately the same level. (Click on the IClamp diamond in the Stimulus Control panel to gain access to the parameters of the pulse.)

## 2. Run the simulation

What are the new values of the initial voltage, the voltage at 1/e of the initial voltage, and the length constant? How does this value of length constant compare with your original measurement? It should be <u>twice as large</u>.

## 3. Reset all parameters to their default values

## DOES THE LENGTH CONSTANT CHANGE WITH CHANGES IN MEMBRANE CAPACITANCE?

### 1. Why change the capacitance?

There are two cell types in which the capacitance of a cell changes due to cell structure. The first is the myelinated axon, where each unit area of axonal membrane has a considerably lower capacitance due to the membrane wrappings of the myelin (capacitors in series); the second is the muscle fiber, where each unit area of muscle membrane has a sixfold higher capacitance because of the invaginating membrane of the T-tubule system. How do changes in capacitance affect voltage spread in these cells?

### 2. Change the capacitance and re-run the simulation

Change the capacitance by a factor of, say, two. Does the length constant <u>change</u>?

### 3. Reset the membrane capacitance to its default value

Click on the red box.

## MOVE THE STIMULATING ELECTRODE AND OBSERVE THE PATTERNS OF VOLTAGE SPREAD

Note that the ends of this axon are "sealed"—that is, they have infinite resistance. The voltage change near the end of an axon is especially affected by the resistance of the end. (This will be obvious when you move the electrode towards an end, as suggested in step #3 below).

### 1. Move the electrode (blue ball) to the middle of the axon

Do this in the Stimulus Control panel by clicking on the midpoint of the line representing the axon. Read the new location of the electrode just above the white lower window; it should be at the (0.5) position.

### 2. Stimulate the axon at its midpoint

Click R&R. Note how the voltage spread now <u>differs</u> from the pattern when the electrode was located at the left end of the axon.

### 3. *Move the electrode closer to one end than the other, (e.g., 0.25 or 0.75)*

Because the axon has been divided into 101 short segments for simulation, you will not be able to locate these points precisely but you can get very close (e.g., 0.252475). Stimulate the cell at this asymmetric point.

Observe the voltage decay away from the the point of current injection in the Voltage-vs-Space plot. The pattern of decay is quite different in the two directions.

### 4. *Question*

<u>Why</u> is there no voltage decay at the very ends of the axon (seen earliest at the end nearest the current injection)?

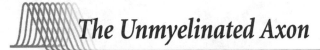

# The Unmyelinated Axon

## Experiment with the Impulse Traveling in the Classic Giant Axon of the Squid

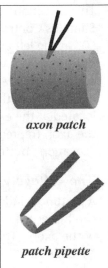

*axon patch*

*patch pipette*

**In this tutorial you will begin studying the propagating action potential.**
The simulations here are of impulses propagating in the squid's giant axon, truly a giant at 500 μm in diameter. By comparison, mammalian unmyelinated fibers, which carry sensations of pain and temperature, are less than 1 μm in diameter. The squid axon has provided neurobiologists with a wonderful experimental preparation.

**Why is the squid axon's diameter so large?**
You will see in this tutorial that rapid propagation of the impulse along an unmyelinated nerve requires that the axon's diameter be large. In mammals, most axons are wrapped with myelin to increase the speed of propagation without having to increase fiber diameter (as you will see in the <u>Myelinated Axon</u> tutorial). In mammals, unmyelinated axons carry sensations that do not require action in the sub-second time frame.

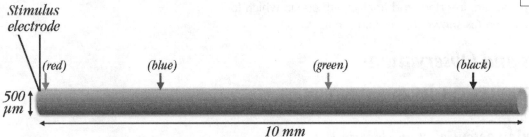

## Goals of this Tutorial
• To understand the mechanisms that underlie propagation of the action potential along the axon
• To relate the shape of the action potential as a function of time to its shape as a function of space
• To observe the effects of changing diameter and temperature on the shape and velocity of the propagating action potential

## Start the Simulation

Click this button to bring up the panels and windows of the simulation.

**Start the Simulation**

# Description of the Panels and Windows Customized for this Tutorial

### 1. Assumptions

This tutorial assumes that you are familiar with the panels and manipulations of *NIA*. Consult the "Help with..." links on the side bar if you need assistance.

### 2. The stimulating electrode

The "Location" of the stimulating electrode (blue ball) is represented in the Stimulus Control panel as the fraction of the distance along the axon from "0" at the left end to "1" at the right end (as it was in the Passive Axon tutorial). As shown in the diagram here, the electrode is located at the extreme left end of the axon (represented below the "Location" button as "axon[0]").

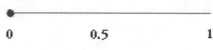

### 3. The Voltage-vs-Time graph

A plotting window comes up automatically in which the action potential can be recorded by an electrode inserted into the center (the 0.5 position) of the axon. (This location of the recording site is printed on the graph as "axon.v[0.5].") During the tutorial, this graph will be overlaid with one in which two electrodes are inserted, and finally, with one in which four electrodes are inserted (as shown in the diagram above).

# Experiments and Observations

## RECORD THE ACTION POTENTIAL AS A FUNCTION OF TIME AT VARIOUS LOCATIONS ALONG THE AXON

### 1. Record the action potential at one location

Press R&R. The axon is stimulated at its left end and the action potential is recorded at the center of the axon. Would you see a similar recording if you stimulated the axon at its right end? Do the experiment: Move the electrode by clicking on the line at the right end. (Please move it back afterwards for the next experiment.)

### 2. Observe the currents and conductances underlying the propagating action potential

Press the "Membrane Currents" and "Membrane Conductances" buttons to bring up graphs in which you can view the Na and K currents and conductances at the center of the axon. Run the simulation and look carefully at the temporal relations of the voltage, currents, and conductances.

### 3. Questions

Do the ionic current patterns for this propagating action potential appear similar to those for an action potential in a uniform patch, which you observed in the Na Action Potential tutorial? You will see below that the advancing impulse propagates because of the longitudinal currents that flow from the impulse to depolarize the membrane ahead. <u>How can it be</u>, then, that the currents in a *propagating* impulse at any given point in the axon have time courses similar to those for a *stationary* impulse in a patch?

### 4. *Record the action potential at two locations*

Close the Membrane Currents and Membrane Conductances graphs. Press the "Voltage vs Time, Dual traces" button; the graph you call up will overlie the previous graph. Two recording electrodes are now inserted, located near the two ends of the axon (locations 0.1 and 0.9). Since the stimulating electrode is located at the left end, the action potential will arrive earlier at the red recording electrode than at the black one. Run the simulation. Move the stimulating electrode to the right end of the axon and run the simulation again. Move it back, for the next experiment.

### 5. *Record the action potential at four locations*

Press the "Voltage vs Time, Quad traces" button, then R&R, to do this experiment with four recording electrodes spaced along the axon at positions 0.01, 0.3, 0.6, and 0.9. From these plots, see if you can envision the membrane potential distribution as a function of space. This mental task is not easy. Here is where computer simulations can really show off their potential as visual aids to understanding.

### 6. *Prepare to see a movie of the impulse propagating*

Close the Membrane Currents and Membrane Conductances windows. Leave open the Membrane Voltage-vs-Time (Single Trace) plot.

## DISPLAY THE IMPULSE AS IT TRAVELS ALONG THE AXON (VOLTAGE AS A FUNCTION OF SPACE)

### 1. *Bring up the Voltage-vs-Space graph*

Notice that the axon is 10,000 μm (10 mm) long; the four locations at which the voltage is recorded as a function of time are indicated as colored arrows along the *x*-axis. If you re-open the Voltage-vs-Time Quad Traces graph you will observe traces that are color-coded to these arrows.

### 2. *Press R&R to run the movie*

You will generate an action potential with a depolarizing current pulse at the left end of the axon and see the impulse propagate from left to right. You may be surprised by what you see: The voltage distribution is almost uniform along the axon! (You can use the slider in the Run Control panel to control the speed of the simulation.)

### 3. *Relate what you see in the movie to the Voltage-vs-Time plots*

- Stop the action potential about halfway through its travel and be certain you know where its rising phase is on the Voltage-vs-Space plot. You may have to think twice about this because of your familiarity with the rising phase in the Voltage-vs-Time plots.

- Try to follow the voltage at one spatial point as it moves up and down with time.

### 4. Follow the action potential in an advance-pause manner

- First press Reset (not Reset and Run) in Run Control.

- Then press the "Continue for (ms)" button to advance the movie in brief time increments, for example 0.1 ms. Each time you press this button, the movie will advance another 0.1 ms and pause.

## OBSERVE THE EFFECT OF CHANGING THE AXON DIAMETER ON IMPULSE PROPAGATION

### 1. Select Keep Lines in the Membrane Voltage-vs-Time (single trace) graph

With the right mouse button and the cursor on the graph, select the Keep Lines feature so that you can compare the shapes of action potentials generated with different axon diameters.

### 2. Open the Axon Parameters panel to change the diameter

By how much must you reduce the diameter of the axon so that you can see more of its waveform in the movie? When you reduce the diameter, why can you see more of its waveform?

As the axon diameter is decreased, less current is necessary to stimulate it. (Why is this?) The current, then, may be reduced to minimize the current "shock artifact" during the stimulus by selecting IClamp in the Stimulus Control panel and reducing the amplitude of the current pulse from 20,000 nA to a lower value.

### 3. Question

In the Voltage-vs-Time graph, notice what happens to the delay of the action potential with respect to the stimulus, and also whether the shape of the action potential is affected when the axon's diameter is changed over two log units. Can you explain your observations?

### 4. Prepare for the next experiments

Restore the default diameter and erase the Voltage-vs-Time traces. Continue to Keep Lines.

## OBSERVE THE EFFECT OF CHANGES IN TEMPERATURE ON THE PROPAGATION OF THE IMPULSE

### 1. Warm the axon by 5°C

Store the Voltage-vs-Time traces with Keep Lines. How is the action potential affected? Click here for a discussion.

### 2. Continue to increase the temperature in 5°C steps

As you increase the temperature, do you find a point where the action potential fails? Exactly how does it fail, and why? Click here for the answer.

### 3. Restore the default temperature to prepare for the next experiment

## MEASURE THE VELOCITY OF PROPAGATION OF THE IMPULSE

### 1. *How does one measure velocity experimentally?*

Two electrodes are inserted into the axon a known distance apart, and the time at which the impulse crosses some chosen voltage is measured at each location. The velocity may then be calculated since velocity is equal to the distance between the electrodes divided by the time it takes for the impulse to travel from one electrode to the next (mm/sec). You can do this with the Voltage-vs-Time, Dual Traces graph, using the crosshairs to measure the time at which each action potential crosses zero.

### 2. *Call up the Voltage-vs-Time, Dual Traces graph and measure velocity*

Using the difference in the time of zero-crossing for the impulse at each of these recording sites, and the 8000 μm length between them, calculate the impulse conduction velocity (velocity = length/time). You will have to put up with a certain amount of imprecision due to the time resolution of the points plotting the action potentials.

### 3. *Measure the velocity as a function of axon diameter*

For small diameters you may notice that the action potential is so slow that it does not pass the 0.9 position in the 5 ms allotted on the graph. You can set the Total # (ms) (in Run Control) to a greater value (e.g., 10 ms). Remember to decrease the amplitude of the stimulus current as you decrease diameter.

Keep your plot of velocity versus diameter for comparison with a similar plot you will make in the next tutorial for the myelinated nerve. There is a critical diameter below which myelination confers no advantage. You will be able to determine this value.

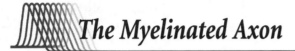# *The Myelinated Axon*

## How Impulses Can Travel at 50 Miles per Hour!

**The sciatic nerve of the frog is the classic preparation for myelinated axons in vertebrates.**
In this tutorial you will simulate high-speed impulse propagation in a single, myelinated axon of the frog. You may find features of impulse conduction in myelinated nerve surprisingly different from descriptions in some textbooks.

**Notice the axon's small diameter compared to that of the squid axon.**
The frog axon's diameter is typically 10 μm rather than the squid's extraordinary 500 μm. In spite of the 50-fold reduction in its diameter, the many wraps of the membrane making up the myelin boost the frog axon's velocity to rival that of the squid! In mammals, the smallest myelinated fibers are a little less than 1 μm.

**The simulated axon has ten myelinated regions (internodes).**
Each internode is 1000 μm (1 mm) long. Between each internode, and at the two ends of the axon, are the nodes, each 3.2 μm long. Thus the axon's total length is 10,035 μm, marginally longer than that of the squid axon in <u>The Unmyelinated Axon</u> tutorial. Notice that the nodes make an insignificant contribution to the axon's total length.

**How are ion channels distributed in the axonal membrane of myelinated axons?**
Myelination alters the axonal <u>distribution of channels</u>. Within the <u>myelinated regions</u>, the normal Hodgkin-Huxley ion-channel densities have been assigned for these simulations. At the nodes, the densities are tenfold greater than normal, matching <u>experimental observations</u> and <u>simulation analysis</u>.

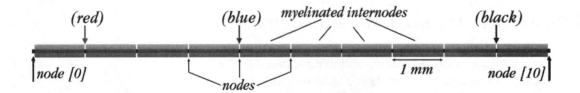

### Goals of this Tutorial
- To observe that the impulse does not "jump" from node to node but spreads out, covering many nodes at once
- To measure the velocity of impulse propagation in myelinated nerve and compare it to unmyelinated nerve
- To change the degree of myelination and the temperature—two clinically important factors—and observe the effect on conduction velocity

## Start the Simulation

Click this button to bring up the panels and windows of the simulation.

> **Start the Simulation**

## Description of the Panels and Windows Customized for this Tutorial

### 1. The stimulating electrode

The stimulating electrode is located in the center (0.5) of node[0], the node at the extreme left end of the axon. This location is specified as node[0](0.5), just above the lower portion of the Stimulus Control panel.

### 2. The graphs

Launch the Voltage-vs-Time and Voltage-vs-Space graphs when called for in the tutorial steps. The color-coded, voltage-recording electrodes are located as shown in the diagram above.

### 3. The parameters panels

The Nodal and Myelinated Region Parameters panels are read-out only; you should not attempt to change the numbers in the fields as changes will have no effect on the simulation. The values for capacitance, leakage, and channel density in the Myelinated Region panel will be calculated and displayed according to the number of myelin wraps.

## Experiments and Observations

### OBSERVE THE SHAPE OF THE IMPULSE IN A MYELINATED AXON

### 1. Record the action potential at node[4]

Observe the action potential in the Voltage-vs-Time, Single-trace graph. When you run the simulation, you will record the action potential in the middle (0.5) of node[4].

### 2. Press Node Currents (P&G Manager) to view INa and IK at node[4]

Is there any marked difference in shape, timing, or amplitude between the currents flowing into the node and the currents you observed underlying the action potential in the Unmyelinated Axon tutorial? Should there be?

### OBSERVE IMPULSE PROPAGATION IN A MYELINATED AXON

### 1. Call up the Voltage-vs-Space graph and run the simulation

The impulse will propagate along the axon from the stimulating electrode, at the left end, to the right. Are you surprised by its peculiar ratchet-like appearance? Use the "Stop" button to freeze the action potential and examine these bumps more closely. Are they real or an artifact of doing experiments with a simulator?

Remember that you can also pause the movie at selected intervals by clicking Reset, then the "Continue for (ms)" button, typing the interval in the field of this button.

## 2. *Record the impulse at nodes [1], [4], and [9]*

Call up the Voltage-vs-Time, Dual Traces graph. It will overlie the Node Currents graph. Recording electrodes are now located at node[1] and node[9], in addition to the one in the uppermost graph at node[4]. When you run the simulation, make certain that the time at which each electrode records the impulse makes sense.

## MEASURE CONDUCTION VELOCITY AND DETERMINE HOW THE DEGREE OF MYELINATION AFFECTS VELOCITY

### 1. *Use the recording electrodes at nodes[1] and [9] to measure velocity*

As you did in the Unmyelinated Axon tutorial, use the crosshairs to measure the time at which each action potential reaches some reference point; it is best to choose the time at which the rising phase crosses zero. The recording electrodes are 8000 μm apart. Using this information, calculate the velocity.

### 2. *What is the relation between number of myelin wraps and the axon's capacitance and conductance?*

You can change the number of wraps of myelin in the field associated with that button in the P&G Manager. As you change the number of wraps, follow how wrapping affects the membrane's net capacitance and conductance in the Myelinated Region Parameters panel. You will need to adjust the stimulus amplitude as the number of wraps is increased. Start with zero wraps and then increase the number, say, by ones or tens. Do not be concerned about the jagged impulse that you see when the number of myelin wraps is small.

When you set the number of myelin wraps to "0," you have an unmyelinated axon so the membrane has a capacitance (Cm) of 1 μF/cm². As you add wraps, the capacitance is reduced to 0.5 μF/cm² with one wrap, to 0.333 μF/cm² with two wraps, etc. The capacitance decreases according to the equation for capacitors in series.

Since the wrapping membrane also has resistance, the effective resistance of the internode region increases in proportion to the number of wraps. Correspondingly, the conductance of the stacked membranes decreases with wrapping (because conductance is the reciprocal of resistance).

### 3. *Now determine the velocity of the impulse as a function of the number of wraps*

Measure and plot (manually) the velocity versus the number of wraps. This experiment should give you an appreciation of the effectiveness of myelin. Does increasing the number of wraps above 150 offer a proportional increase in the velocity of propagation?

### 4. *Restore the number of wraps to the default value of 150*

## WHAT IS THE EFFECT OF
## TEMPERATURE ON THE PROPAGATION VELOCITY?

### 1. Compare the velocity in myelinated frog axon with that in unmyelinated squid axon

Do the small, myelinated axons of frogs conduct at roughly the same velocity as the unmyelinated huge axons of squids? To compare the velocity of myelinated frog axon to the velocity you calculated for the squid axon, cool the myelinated axon to 6.3°C (the temperature for squid axon) and determine the velocity.

By how much is the impulse in myelinated axon slowed when it is cooled from the default temperature of 22°C to 6.3°C?

### 2. Plot the velocity as a function of temperature

Cool and warm the myelinated axon by increments or decrements of 5 or 10°C. This experiment assumes that you have already experimented with the effects of changing temperature on the action potential in the Na Action Potential tutorial and the Unmyelinated Axon tutorial. If you have not, and you wish to know more about the effect of temperature on the action potential, consult this link.

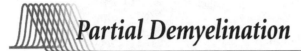

# Partial Demyelination

## The Problem in Multiple Sclerosis

**This tutorial simulates the condition of multiple sclerosis.**
This tutorial simulates an action potential in myelinated nerve attempting to propagate through a demyelinated (bare) region, as in multiple sclerosis (MS). In this disease, axons become demyelinated in a patchy and unpredictable fashion, leading to a host of sensory and motor symptoms.

**The preparation is demyelinated on the left half.**
The axon is 10,000 µm long, as shown in the diagram below. The right half is myelinated, with 5 node/myelinated internode pairs; the left half is demyelinated. You can change parameters both for the bare half and for the myelinated half. In the tutorial you will first insert a stimulating electrode into the left end of the bare axon, then move it to the right end of the myelinated region (node[4]).

**How are channels distributed in the membrane of a demyelinated axon?**
Ion channel densities have been assigned on the basis of experimental observations. The densities in the nodes are tenfold greater than those in squid axon. The bare axon has been assigned the normal density of channels in unmyelinated nerve, distributed uniformly. The distribution of channels in demyelinated axon is only <u>partially understood</u> at present and depends on how long the axon has been demyelinated.

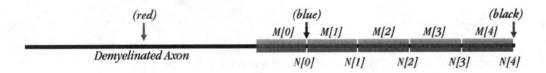

**Goals of this Tutorial**
- To observe the shape of the action potential as it travels from the demyelinated region of the axon into the myelinated region
- To observe the features of the action potential as it tries to invade the bare axon from the myelinated region
- To observe how changes in the ion conductances in the bare axon and also in temperature affect the ability of the action potential to invade the bare axon from the myelinated portion

## Start the Simulation

Click this button to bring up the panels and windows of the simulation.

[ Start the Simulation ]

## Description of the Panels and Windows Customized for this Tutorial

### 1. Assumptions

This tutorial assumes that you are now familiar with the following panels and manipulations:

- The function of the buttons within the P&G Manager and Run Control panels

- Running simulations by clicking Reset and Run (R&R) or clicking Reset and then the "Continue for (ms)" button in the Run Control panel

- Inserting stimulating electrodes by launching the Stimulus Control panel and controlling the onset, amplitude, and duration of the stimulus

- Storing, erasing, resizing, and measuring values on traces in plotting windows using the right mouse button features

- Using the field editor or the arrows box to change values in the parameters panels

If this tutorial is your introduction to *Neurons in Action*, we suggest that you familiarize yourself with the panels and operations listed here by clicking their links.

### 2. The stimulating electrodes

Two "Stimulus Control" buttons are available in the P&G Manager, one to put the stimulating electrode (Stimulus 'Trode) in the left end of the bare axon (brought up initially) and the other to put it in the right end (node[4]) of the myelinated segment. Clicking either of these buttons will bring up separate Stimulus Control panels.

Although the electrode may be moved after insertion as usual by clicking on the line representing the axon in this panel, it is preferable to switch locations using the Stimulus Control buttons because the amplitude of the current stimulus needs to be different in the bare axon and in the myelinated segment.

### 3. The graphs

In the Voltage-vs-Time graph, the traces are color-coded to the three recording sites shown in the diagram above and on the axis of the Voltage-vs-Space graph:

- At the center of the bare half of the axon (red)

- At node[0] (blue)

- At node[4] (black)

# Experiments and Observations

## OBSERVE IMPULSES TRAVELING IN PARTIALLY DEMYELINATED AXONS

### 1. Stimulate the left end of the demyelinated (bare) axon

- **Observe the location of the stimulating electrode.**
  The Stimulus Control panel that comes up upon launching the simulation shows a stimulating electrode in the left end of the bare half of the axon. The amplitude of the current pulse has been set to a large enough value to evoke an action potential in the bare portion.

- **Run the simulation (press R&R)**
  The impulse will be initiated at the far-left end of the demyelinated region and travel to the right into the myelinated region.

  In the Voltage-vs-Time graph, notice that the second and third recorded impulses (recorded at the nodes) are much closer together than are the first and second recorded impulses (recorded in the bare area and at the first node). <u>Why is this</u>?

- **Relate the Voltage-vs-Time recordings to the Voltage-vs-Space movie.**
  As you did in the <u>Unmyelinated Axon</u> tutorial, watch the voltage at a point in the Voltage-vs-Space graph as it moves up and down in time. If you pick a point where a recording electrode is located (for example, in the middle of the bare axon), you can compare it to the trace in the Voltage-vs-Time graph.

  To slow down the process, click the "Continue for (ms)" button in the Run Control panel to play and pause the movie repeatedly. Or click the "Stop" button to stop the movie at any time.

- **Stop the impulse in the bare axon.**
  Make certain you understand the shape of the action potential in both plots. For example, which phase is the rising phase in the Voltage-vs-Time plot and in the Voltage-vs-Space plot? Can you explain the <u>shape of the rising phase</u> in the Voltage-vs-Space plot? If you understand the shape, you probably have a good understanding of how the impulse propagates.

- **Close the Stimulus 'Trode in Bare Axon panel.**
  This action will remove the stimulating electrode. You will next insert it at the other end of the axon. Although you can move the electrode to the other end of the axon by clicking on the line, the amplitude of the stimulus will then be inappropriately large for stimulating the myelinated segment, as mentioned above.

  **ATTENTION!** *Next you will put the stimulating electrode in node[4]. It is necessary to close the Stimulus 'Trode in Bare Axon panel to avoid generating impulses at both ends of the axon.*

### 2. Reverse the direction of stimulation: Excite the myelinated region

Press Stimulus 'Trode in Node[4] to insert the stimulating electrode at the rightmost node of the myelinated region. Run the simulation. What happens to the impulse at the junction between the myelinated and bare axon? Explain your observations. Relate what you see in the Voltage-vs-Space movie to your recordings with the three electrodes in the Voltage-vs-Time graph.

### A CHANGE IN TEMPERATURE IS KNOWN TO IMPROVE THE CONDITION OF MULTIPLE SCLEROSIS PATIENTS. INVESTIGATE THE BASIS FOR THIS PHENOMENON

#### 1. Make an educated guess

Would you expect warming or cooling to improve the prospects of impulse invasion of the demyelinated region? Recall your experiments on the effect of temperature on the Na action potential.

Hint: What change will enable the action potential in the myelinated segment to supply more current to the bare axon?

#### 2. Test your hypothesis

Change the temperature (in the Run Control panel). Run the simulation to see if impulse invasion of the demyelinated region improves or worsens. A detailed discussion of the connection between temperature, threshold, and impulse propagation is available.

(Although the temperature range in which you are experimenting is appropriate for frog axon and not for humans, the principle is the same for both species.)

#### 3. Question

What is the smallest change in temperature required to produce any difference you observe? Your observations have a clinical correlation in the Uhthoff phenomenon.

#### 4. Observe impulse resurgence in the myelinated axon

Note that at a certain critical temperature the conditions are just right for the impulse to resurge in the myelinated region; in the Voltage-vs-Time graph you should be able to see two action potential peaks at node[4] (black trace).

#### 5. Restore the temperature to the default value of 25.2°C

### WHAT CHANGES IN AXON PARAMETERS WILL PERMIT THE IMPULSE TO INVADE THE BARE REGION?

#### 1. Launch the Bare Axon Parameters panel

In this panel you can alter parameters of the demyelinated portion of the axon. When you have changed a parameter, remember to reset it before changing another one. You can experiment with changes that will promote impulse invasion of the bare axon.

- **Change the density of functional K channels.**
  For a hint, read a quote from the National Institutes of Health web page entitled "Therapy to improve nerve impulse conduction."

- **Change the density of functional Na channels.**
  By how much must you change the density to enable invasion of the bare axon?

- **Change the diameter of the bare axon.**
  In what direction would you expect a change to facilitate impulse invasion?

  Hint: Changing the diameter of the bare axon changes the membrane area and thus the capacitance that the current from the myelinated axon is required to charge.

- **Prepare for the next experiments.**
  Be certain to restore all bare axon parameters to their default values. You can close the Bare Axon Parameters panel or leave it open.

## 2. Change parameters of the myelinated axon

Click the "Internode Parameters" button. Four menus will come up in a "tray" for four of the five internodes (M[0] through M[3] on the diagram above). The far right internode, M[4], is left out. You can adjust the length of each internode, its degree of myelination (the capacitance, which is $1 \ \mu F/cm^2$ divided by the number of wraps), and the inside diameter of the axon (the diameter of the axon without its wrapping).

- **Experiment with the internode M[0].**
  What change in the parameters of this adjacent internode will increase the longitudinal current into the bare axon and cause the action potential to propagate there?

  - Questions: What if you <u>change the length</u> of this myelinated segment? Should it be longer or shorter to supply more current to the bare axon? How much change is needed?

  - Question: What if you <u>change the degree of myelination</u> of this segment by changing the capacitance?

  - Question: Will <u>changing the diameter</u> of this one internode have an effect? Hint: Any change that increases the longitudinal current supplied to the bare region of axon from the myelinated region will assist the struggling action potential to become regenerative.

- **Change parameters of the other internodes.**
  How crucial is the adjacent internode compared to the more remote internodes? Experiment in a similar fashion with the other three internodes.

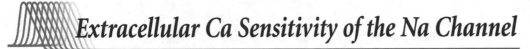# *Extracellular Ca Sensitivity of the Na Channel*

## Abnormal Serum [Ca] Can Cause Clinical Hypo- and Hyperexcitability

**[Ca]o levels affect the excitability of nerve and muscle.**
This tutorial will demonstrate the remarkable sensitivity of the Na channel to the concentration of Ca in the serum or bathing medium. Raising the [Ca]o has a "stabilizing" effect on nerve and muscle excitability, as was observed by a number of investigators during the decades preceding the Hodgkin-Huxley papers. Lowering the [Ca]o has the opposite effect, making the nerve and muscle hyperexcitable. Both effects come about through the direct action of Ca on ion channels, particularly the Na channel.

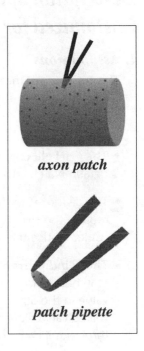

*axon patch*

*patch pipette*

**Major clinical problems can result when serum [Ca] deviates from its normal levels.**
When Ca levels in the serum are too high (hypercalcemia), a patient typically has symptoms resulting from the decreased excitability of neurons: fatigue, depression, confusion, and cardiac arrhythmias. In extreme cases, coma and death can result. Ca levels that are too low (hypocalcemia) result in symptoms of increased excitability: cardiac arrhythmias, cramps, tingling in the extremities, interruption of breathing because of spasms of the larynx or bronchial tubes, or even seizures. While extracellular Ca homeostasis can be affected by a variety of disorders, hypocalcemia often results from hypoparathyroidism.

**How does the [Ca]o affect membrane excitability?**
In the Voltage Clamping a Patch tutorial, by looking at families of currents, you explored the exquisite voltage sensitivity of the Na and K channels that was revealed by Hodgkin and Huxley's 1952 experiments. Hodgkin, working with Frankenhauser, went on to discover that external Ca actually shifts the voltage sensitivity for both channel types. Subsequent attempts to understand the precise action of Ca are detailed in Chapter 20 of *Ion Channels in Excitable Membranes,* 3rd Ed. by Hille (2001).

**In this tutorial you can experiment with the action of [Ca]o on the Na channel.**
These simulations use the Moore-Cox (MC) model of the Na channel, which incorporates Ca acting directly on one of the closed states of the channel.

**Goals of this Tutorial**
• To understand how the [Ca]o can influence excitability by affecting the Na channel
• To explore the basis of spontaneous firing in conditions of low [Ca]o

## Start the Simulation

Click this button to bring up the panels and windows of the simulation.

**Start the Simulation**

## Description of the Panels and Windows Customized for this Tutorial

### 1. Assumptions

This tutorial assumes that you have completed the <u>Threshold</u> and <u>Voltage Clamping a Patch</u> tutorials.

### 2. The Panel & Graph Manager

- **The "HH Na channel" button:** This button runs the simulations with the default Na channels that are not Ca-sensitive.

- **The "MooreCox (MC) Na channel" button:** By clicking this button you replace the HH Na channels with MC Na channels that are sensitive to the [Ca]o. Notice the changes in the "Patch Parameters" panel.

- **The "Find Current Threshold" button:** This button, when pressed, searches for the amplitude of the stimulus current at threshold. Read this value in the Stimulus Control panel (IClamp mode, amplitude field). There will be variability from trial to trial in the precise value of the current beyond three significant figures.

### 3. The Patch Parameters panel

When the HH Na channels are being simulated, the conductance of the Ca-sensitive MC Na channel is zero and vice versa. You may vary the [Ca]o, but the simulations may not be realistic for levels of [Ca]o below 0.5 mM for the MC Na channels.

### 4. The graphs

Graphs display membrane voltage and Na current. Na currents plotted with the HH Na channels are red and those plotted with MC Na channels are green.

## Experiments and Observations

### COMPARE ACTION POTENTIALS GENERATED BY HH AND MC Na CHANNELS

Before experimenting with the effect of [Ca]o on the channels, you should assure yourself that the equations for the MC Na channels simulate action potentials that closely match those simulated by the HH equations when [Ca]o is at its normal value of 2 mM.

### 1. Click R&R to generate the normal action potential and INa

Keep Lines in the the "Voltage vs Time"and "Na Current vs Time" graphs to compare these traces with those generated by the MC Na channels in the next step.

### 2. Click the "MooreCox (MC) Na Channel" button

Be sure the conductances have changed in the "Patch Parameters" panel, and then press R&R. Notice that there is a slight difference between the two action potentials and their underlying currents: The MC action potential falls off relatively smoothly while the HH action potential displays an "anomalous hump."

## EXPERIMENT WITH CHANGING [Ca]o

### 1. Assure yourself that the HH action potential is insensitive to [Ca]o

Return to the HH Na channels. Change the [Ca]o, using Keep Lines to compare action potentials generated at each concentration. (Yes, this experiment is boring; controls often are.) Erase lines to prepare for more interesting experiments.

### 2. Substitute the MC Na channels for the HH Na channels, then change [Ca]o

- **Increase the [Ca]o to 3 mM to mimic hypercalcemia.**
  Raised [Ca]o in the serum causes symptoms indicative of decreased excitability of cells. Is the patch now indeed less excitable? If so, what can you do to generate an action potential?

- **Decrease the [Ca]o to 1 mM to mimic hypocalcemia.**
  Lowered [Ca]o in the serum leads to symptoms of increased excitability of cells. What changes do you observe in the action potential and Na current caused by changing [Ca]o from 2 mM to 1 mM? Do your results indicate increased membrane excitability?

### 3. Observe the effect of [Ca]o on the Na current in voltage clamp

- **In Stimulus Control, click VClamp.**
  Using the default settings, observe the effect of changing [Ca]o on the INa. Are your results similar to what you would predict if [Ca]o shifted the voltage dependence of the channel?

- **Return to IClamp for the next experiments.**

## MIGHT THE PATCH BE FIRING SPONTANEOUSLY IN 1 mM [Ca]o?

Most neurons require a stimulus current of some type to excite them into generating an action potential. This current might be postsynaptic current resulting from the opening of transmitter-gated channels, or current flowing in advance of a propagating action potential to bring the next portion of an axon to threshold, or current injected by the experimenter through an electrode. Some neurons—pacemakers, or neurons in an abnormal state—fire spontaneously without a stimulus current.

### 1. Check for spontaneous firing

- **Increase the Total # (ms) in Run Control to, say, 50 ms or more.**
  To check for spontaneous firing, you will want a longer time base.

- **In IClamp, set the amplitude of the current stimulus to zero.**

- **Re-run the simulation at 1 m*M* [Ca]o.**
  What happens to the action potential and Na current when you lower
  [Ca]o to 0.9 or 0.8 m*M*? (Reminder: the MC model may not be accurate
  below 0.5 m*M* [Ca]o.)

2. ***When a neuron fires spontaneously, where is its threshold?***
   In the <u>Threshold</u> tutorial, you saw that the current required to trigger an HH
   action potential had a precise value. How does Ca binding to the MC Na
   channel influence the value of this threshold current?

   - **Find the value of the stimulus threshold current (in nA) for
     2 m*M* [Ca]o.**
     To do this, click the "Find Current Threshold" button instead of R&R to
     run the simulation. Record the displayed value.

   - **Next, find the threshold in 3 m*M* [Ca]o.**
     Does the amplitude of the threshold current in elevated [Ca]o make sense
     in terms of your observations (above) on the action potential?

   - **Now, attempt to find the threshold current amplitude for
     1 m*M* [Ca]o.**
     Can you explain your observation? What is the <u>meaning of "threshold"</u> for
     this spontaneous action potential?

   - **Compare spontaneous and triggered impulses.**
     Using Keep Lines, compare a spontaneous impulse in 1 m*M* [Ca]o with a
     subthreshold response and a suprathreshold impulse generated in 2 m*M*
     [Ca]o. Are you convinced that the spontaneous action potential does not
     have a threshold? Look at the rates of rise of all three traces.

3. ***For a deeper understanding of excitability, threshold, and
   spontaneous firing, proceed to the next tutorial, the <u>Dynamic
   View of Threshold</u>***

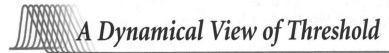

# A Dynamical View of Threshold

## The Rate of Change of the Voltage Determines Firing

### What is threshold?

Threshold is such an important concept in neuroscience that it is essential to attempt to define it precisely. There is a rich <u>history</u> of neuroscientists attempting to understand threshold. The <u>Threshold</u> tutorial showed that threshold is *not* a fixed voltage. What, then, is threshold?

### In this tutorial you will measure the *rate of change* of the voltage before the impulse takes off.

Usually voltage (Vm) is plotted versus time. But here we ask: What is the rate of change of the voltage—the slope—just below and just above threshold? Is there a particular rate of change that constitutes threshold?

### Goals of this Tutorial

- To refine the definition of threshold by observing the rate of depolarization (dV/dt) of the membrane
- To become acquainted with an informative way of plotting the dynamics of the action potential: as dV/dt versus the voltage (Vm) (known in physics and engineering as a "phase plane" plot)
- To explore the factors that can affect the value of the threshold dV/dt

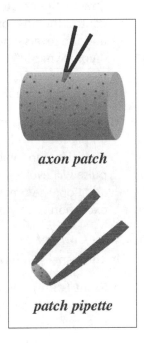

*axon patch*

*patch pipette*

## Start the Simulation

Click this button to bring up the panels and windows of the simulation.

> **Start the Simulation**

## Description of the Panels and Windows Customized for this Tutorial

### 1. A new set of graphs: dV/dt versus Voltage

Beneath the Voltage-vs-Time window is a graph that plots the rate of change of voltage (dV/dt, ordinate, or *y*-axis) versus the voltage during the action potential (abscissa, or *x*-axis). Two additional graphs may be launched from the P&G Manager to view this plot at a higher resolution.

### 2. The Panel & Graph Manager

- **dV/dt vs Voltage, Medium Resolution:** The scale chosen for this graph should allow you to view the entire stimulus pulse or synaptic potential.

- **dV/dt vs Voltage, High Resolution:** Clicking this button brings up a graph—on top of the Medium Resolution graph—that plots the slope of the voltage change with a very high resolution. Each time either the Medium or High Resolution button is clicked, the graphs appear on top of the existing dV/dt graph.

- **AlphaSynapse:** This button calls up an <u>AlphaSynapse panel</u>, which provides a postsynaptic conductance increase that causes a current to flow that generates an excitatory postsynaptic potential (EPSP). You can control the time of onset, the time to peak (Tpeak), the amplitude (gmax) and the reversal potential (e) of the conductance increase. Pressing the "AlphaSynapse" button also sets the amplitude of the current through the electrode (in Stimulus Control) to zero so that excitation occurs only by way of the synaptic input.

- **Hyperpolarization:** Clicking this button sets values of duration and amplitude for a hyperpolarizing pulse in the Stimulus Control panel, mimicking an inhibitory postsynaptic potential (IPSP). The offset of this pulse will evoke an action potential. It also sets the Total # (ms) to 25. In addition, the gmax (mS) in the AlphaSynapse panel is set to zero so that excitation is only by way of the off-response.

### 3. Run Control

In this panel you have two options for running the simulations:

- **Reset & Run:** Clicking this button runs the simulation at a slow pace that allows you to see how the action potential's dV/dt is plotted as its voltage changes.

- **Reset & Fast Run:** Clicking this button runs the simulation very quickly. It is especially useful when trying different parameter values in an attempt to find threshold precisely.

## Experiments and Observations

### PLOT dV/dt VERSUS Vm DURING SUBTHRESHOLD AND SUPRATHRESHOLD STIMULI

### 1. First, take time to get oriented to this new way of looking at the action potential

We start with the default stimulus current set just below threshold.

- **Examine the subthreshold voltage trace, paying attention to its slope, dV/dt.**
  Notice that Vm lingers near threshold for about 8 ms, rising slowly, then rather abruptly returns to the resting value. During this 8 ms period, dV/dt is rather constant and positive; when Vm returns to rest, actually undershooting the resting value, dV/dt is, of course, negative.

- **Examine the subthreshold slope (dV/dt) in the dV/dt-vs-Voltage plot.**
  Examine the unfamiliar, perhaps even frightening, trace in the plot just below the Voltage-vs-Time window. Initially, there is a huge, positive-going stimulus/plotting artifact. Then the trace is rather flat, an apparently unchanging value of dV/dt, moving from –65 mV to –60 mV. This flat part

represents the steep, depolarizing ramp of voltage increase during the stimulating current step. Before interpreting the rest of the trace, examine it at a higher resolution.

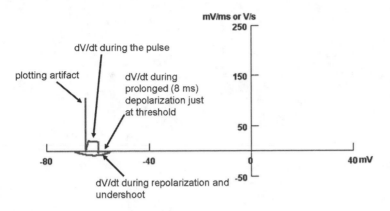

- **Click the "dV/dt-vs-V, Medium Resolution" button to see the events in more detail.**
  When you run the simulation, you will now see that, during the pulse, the dV/dt is actually slowly declining (from 24.3 to 22.2 mV/ms) as the voltage rises. <u>Why is this</u>?

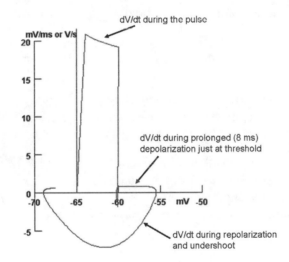

At the end of the pulse, dV/dt drops to a nearly steady level of about 0.95 mV/ms, as the voltage creeps steadily from –60 mV to –56 mV. When the membrane repolarizes, dV/dt becomes negative. Just before the trace ends (at 12 ms on the Voltage-vs-Time plot), the slope once again becomes positive.

- **Increase the stimulus amplitude above threshold.**
  Using the arrows box, increase the stimulus amplitude one tiny step, from 39.518 to 39.519. Observe the action potential in the Voltage-vs-Time plot and in the dV/dt-vs-Voltage plot. In the figure below, we show threshold on the High Resolution graph.

- **Threshold!**
  Select Keep Lines to see that the voltage trajectory of the sub- and supra-threshold stimuli at first follow identical paths with an almost constant

value of dV/dt (about 0.95 mV/ms). Finally, the trajectories diverge when either the Na current becomes large enough to overcome the K current and generate an impulse, or the K current wins, and impulse generation fails.

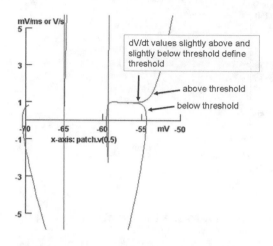

### OBSERVE THE THRESHOLD OF AN ACTION POTENTIAL TRIGGERED BY AN EPSP

Does a natural stimulus, an EPSP, lead to the same sub- and suprathreshold rates of rise as does current injection?

#### 1. Call up the AlphaSynapse panel (from the P&G Manager) to excite the patch with an EPSP

The default stimulus conductance (gmax = 0.59369) is set just subthreshold. Run the simulation, then click the up-arrow to increase the amplitude of the conductance to 0.59370, now above threshold, and run the simulation again.

The synaptic current, due to the conductance increase with its AlphaSynapse kinetics, drives the membrane voltage to the same level as does the square current pulse. Both depolarizations, when near threshold, trigger the "threshold war" between the Na and K currents that persists long after the stimuli are over. Consequently, their stimulus dynamics do not affect the value of the threshold dV/dt.

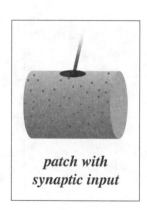

*patch with synaptic input*

### OBSERVE THE THRESHOLD OF AN IMPULSE ARISING AT THE OFFSET OF A HYPERPOLARIZATION (SUCH AS AN IPSP)

An impulse can often arise at the offset of a hyperpolarization that has been caused by injected current or inhibitory transmitter, as you saw in the <u>Synaptic Inhibition</u> tutorial. This phenomenon of increased excitability due to hyperpolarization is called "disinhibition," and the resulting impulse is sometimes called an "off-response." Is the threshold rate of change of the voltage for this impulse the same as that generated by a depolarization?

#### 1. Give a hyperpolarizing pulse that generates an impulse at its offset

• **Click the "Hyperpolarization" button in the P & G Manager.**

   ▪ In the Stimulus Control panel, the pulse duration will be set to 5 ms and its amplitude to –5.8728.

- The Total # (ms) will be set to 25. At threshold, the decision time to fire can be long, so the time base should be increased in order to see any action potential that may occur.

- In the AlphaSynapse menu, the conductance (gmax) will be set to zero so there is no EPSP.

## 2. *Increase the amplitude to above threshold for the off-response*

A slight change (to −5.8729) should work. Now the hyperpolarizing pulse is ever so slightly larger, and the resulting off-response is suprathreshold.

- **Measure the rate of change of the voltage at threshold (the *y*-axis value on the dV/dt-vs-Voltage, High Resolution plot).**
  Is it the same value you measured for injected depolarizing current or for the EPSP? Does the duration of the stimulus matter? (To keep the stimulus at threshold, you must decrease the conductance if you increase the duration of the stimulus.)

## OBSERVE THE THRESHOLD OF SPONTANEOUS
## ACTION POTENTIALS GENERATED BY INCREASING THE [K]o

At the resting potential, there is a small conductance to Na in most neurons, observed in the tutorial on Equilibrium Potentials. Consequently, there is a continuous, small inward Na current balanced by an opposing, small outward K current. When you disturb this balance by increasing the [K]o slightly, making EK slightly less negative, the inward Na current can gain the advantage. Spontaneous action potentials result. How does their threshold rate of rise compare to that of impulses generated by a stimulus at normal [K]o?

## 1. *Set the amplitude of the current stimulus to zero*

In this experiment you will be looking at spontaneous action potentials, not those generated by a stimulus.

## 2. *Leave the time axis at 25 ms*

You will find that, as you suddenly change [K]o at $t = 0$, it may take a long time for the spontaneous action potential to be generated. You do not want to miss an action potential by having too short a time axis. Use Reset & Fast Run in this experiment.

## 3. *Increase the [K]o*

Through successive approximations, we have found the [K]o that is just above and just below threshold. NEURON allows you to specify these concentrations to four decimal places. It may be instructive for you to find these values yourself, and may even be fun as you watch the dV/dt for each concentration on the High Resolution plot. If you would rather jump straight to the answer, however, click this link.

## 4. *Measure the threshold rate of rise for the spontaneous impulse*

You should have measured about 0.8 mV/ms as the threshold rate of rise, a value lower than the 0.95 mV/ms measured for the impulse generated by a stimulus when [K]o was 5 m*M*. Can you explain why the value is lower?

## SHOULD A CHANGE IN TEMPERATURE CHANGE THE VALUE OF THE THRESHOLD RATE OF RISE OF THE ACTION POTENTIAL?

You know that increasing the temperature speeds the kinetics of channel transitions for example, from the closed to the open state at a given depolarization. Higher temperatures will also speed inactivation, in the case of the Na channels. From earlier tutorials you have seen that raising the temperature leads to faster action potentials (which gives us mammals an advantage in brain speed). So you might expect that raising the temperature will lead to a faster rate of rise. But by how much?

### 1. Raise the temperature 10°C to 16.3°C and find the threshold rate of rise

Hodgkin and Huxley found that for a 10°C change in temperature there was a threefold increase in the rate constants for gating the Na and K conductances. Find the <u>threshold current</u> at this temperature, and measure the rate of rise of the action potential. Is it threefold greater than at 6.3°C?

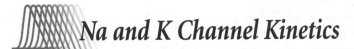

# Na and K Channel Kinetics

## Channel Subtypes, Channel Toxins, Membrane Excitability, and Pain

**The cause of death from eating puffer fish suggests that more than one Na channel type exists.**

Early on, it was known that the toxin in puffer fish—tetrodotoxin (TTX)—caused death from respiratory—rather than cardiac—failure. This distinction indicated that there are differences between the Na channels in nerve and in cardiac muscle. Indeed, it was quickly discovered that some Na channels are resistant to TTX. The subsequent cloning of ion channels in the 80s and 90s revealed a diversity not only in Na channels but in all channel types beyond the wildest speculation.

**Channel subtypes, with their characteristic kinetics, determine neuronal excitability.**

Over 80 genes for subtypes of K channel and nine genes for subtypes of Na channel had been identified in mammals by the beginning of this decade (Hille 2001). Expressed alone, or with other subtypes, these channels determine the excitability of the neuron. Each subtype has its own activation and inactivation kinetics that suit it to its particular job. For a thorough overview of this subject, consult Hille (2001).

**Certain Na channel subtypes have been associated with pathology.**

One example is the Nav1.3 Na channel, which is upregulated in damaged peripheral and central neurons. The kinetics of Nav1.3 cause the neurons that express it to become hyperexcitable, making this channel the likely culprit in neuropathic pain. Mutations in certain other Na channel subtypes change the channel's kinetics, altering membrane excitability and leading to neurological diseases such as epilepsy.

**In this tutorial you can manipulate channel kinetics and observe resulting changes in excitability.**

You can specify the voltage dependence of channel activation and inactivation to mimic different channel subtypes, as well as the action of toxins, that affect channel kinetics. You can then observe the effect of those particular kinetic parameters on membrane excitability.

**Through this tutorial, you should get a "feel" for the HH variables *m*, *n*, and *h*.**

The HH equations include terms that describe the time course and voltage dependence of activation of the Na and K channels and of inactivation of the Na channel. Hodgkin and Huxley selected the letters *m*, *n*, and *h* to represent the probability variables underlying the activation and inactivation processes: *m* and *h* represent activation and inactivation of the Na channel, and *n* represents K channel activation. These variables, which depend on both voltage and time,

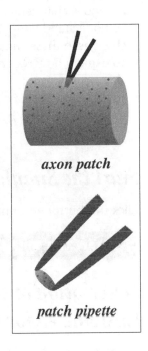

*axon patch*

*patch pipette*

are described by differential equations. The K conductance involves the activation probability, $n$, raised to the fourth power while the Na conductance depends on a product: $h$ multiplied times $m$ cubed. A detailed description of Hodgkin and Huxley's data analysis, and their use of these variables, is available in this link.

**Goals of this Tutorial**
- To appreciate how changes in the activation and inactivation kinetics of the Na and K channels affect membrane excitability
- To understand how $m$, $n$, and $h$ change during the action potential and how changes in these variables affect its shape
- To explore how Na channel subtypes affect excitability through differing channel kinetics
- To observe how Na channel toxins decrease excitability or cause spontaneous firing by altering channel kinetics

# Start the Simulation

Click this button to bring up the panels and windows of the simulation.

> **Start the Simulation**

# Description of the Panels and Windows Customized for this Tutorial

## 1. "Kinetic Parameters Control" button (in the P&G Manager)

This panel, launched by a button in the P&G Manager, has two sections:

- **The left-hand, graphical section:** Three curves are plotted in this graph, each describing probability as a function of voltage:

  - Na channel activation, or "m infinity" ("minf") in black;

  - Na channel inactivation, or "h infinity" ("hinf") in red;

  - K channel activation, or "n infinity" ("ninf") in blue.

- **The right-hand, parameters section:**

  - In the three separate fields, you can change the location of the steady-state values of $m$, $n$, and $h$ along the voltage axis.

  - If you click the box "run after change," the action potential and its underlying currents will be displayed on the graphs after each change, without your having to click R&R.

## 2. "m and h vs Time" and "m, n and h vs Time" buttons (in the P&G Manager)

Each of these buttons launches a graph, overlaying the Current-vs-Time graph, in which the indicated variables are plotted as a function of time during a voltage change.

# Experiments and Observations

## CHANGE THE VOLTAGE SENSITIVITIES OF ACTIVATION OF THE Na AND K CHANNELS

The *m* and *n* relations describe the probabilities that the Na and K channels, respectively, will be activated at a given voltage if that voltage is maintained until these variables reach a steady state.

### 1. *Before you make changes, observe the action potential and its underlying currents with standard HH kinetics*

- **Run the simulation.**
  You should, by now, be very familiar with the shapes of the Na and K currents underlying the action potential. Keep Lines so that in the next experiment you can observe the effects of shifting the Na channel activation curve.

### 2. *Shift the activation (m) curve for the Na channels on the voltage axis in the depolarizing direction*

- **Choose the "vshift-m (mV)" field and, using the arrows box, shift the curve 1 mV in the positive direction.**
  Click the "run after change" box so that the action potential and currents with these new kinetics will be automatically displayed. You should observe that the black *m* curve shifts to the right—the probability of activation of any given Na channel, described by *m*, is now slightly lower. This means that at any given voltage, fewer Na channels are likely to open. Look at the value of *m* at −50 mV, for example, and watch the probability decrease as you shift the curve.

  For a 1 mV shift, what <u>difference</u> in the action potential would you expect to see? Would it be triggered earlier in the pulse (an increase in excitability) or later in the pulse (a decrease in excitability)?

- **Shift the *m* relation another mV in the depolarizing direction.**
  You should now see that the action potential fails altogether. <u>How</u> could you elicit an action potential with the *m* curve shifted?

### 3. *Shift the m relation in the hyperpolarizing direction*

Given the results above, you might expect that shifting the relation in the hyperpolarizing direction would increase excitability and perhaps even lead to spontaneous firing. Does it?

- **Increase the Total # (ms) to 25.**
  Extending the time base will allow you to see any spontaneous action potentials that might occur.

- **Shift *m* gradually in the hyperpolarizing direction, 1 mV at a time.**
  Clearly the membrane has become more excitable. Do you need the stimulus current at all? Set the amplitude of the stimulus current to zero to see if you observe spontaneous firing. If so, by how much did you shift the *m* relation to make the membrane spontaneously excitable?

### 4. Shift the activation relation for the K channels (n)

Since the K current opposes the Na current, you might expect shifts of *n* in the depolarizing direction to increase excitability and shifts in the hyperpolarizing direction to do the opposite. It is instructive to compare a depolarizing shift of 1 mV and 10 mV. What do you <u>observe</u> in the voltage and current plots? Do shifts in *n* also lead to spontaneous firing?

## EXPERIMENT WITH INACTIVATION (h) OF THE Na CHANNEL

The *h* relation describes the probability that channels will *not* be inactivated at a certain voltage. This relation is less confusing if you think of it as the fraction of the Na channels available for opening. That is, at –50 mV only a small fraction of Na channels are available for opening. Notice that at depolarized voltages only a small fraction is available for opening, whereas at very hyperpolarized potentials essentially all of the channels are available (none are inactivated).

### 1. Remove more steady-state inactivation

<u>In which direction</u> would you expect to shift the relation to decrease the number of inactivated channels?

### 2. Push the relation on the voltage axis until you see more than one impulse evoked by the stimulus

By how many mV must you shift the relation to see this evidence of increased excitability?

- **Continue to elicit the first impulse with the stimulus pulse.**
  Extend the time base to 30 ms or more to make sure you are not missing a second action potential.

- **To check for truly spontaneous activity, set the amplitude of the stimulus pulse to zero.**
  Is there a difference between the degree of shift that gives you more than one action potential in response to a stimulus and the degree of shift that permits spontaneous activity? Indeed, <u>why</u> is there spontaneous activity? After all, only the inactivation kinetics have been changed. There has been no change in activation kinetics.

### 3. Shift h in the opposite direction—so that more channels are inactivated at any given voltage

You might expect the impulse to fail as you shift in this direction, but you can overcome this failure by increasing the current. Now, however, the action potential will have a different amplitude and rise time. Can you <u>explain</u> these observations?

### 4. Return the Total # (ms) to its default value of 10 to prepare for the next experiment

## WITH THE VOLTAGE CLAMP, OBSERVE CHANGES IN THE Na AND K CURRENTS WITH SHIFTS IN THE m, n, AND h CURVES

Here, you will voltage clamp the patch, change the voltage dependence of *m*, *n*, and *h*, and observe the changes in the Na and K currents, INa and IK, respectively.

## 1. Voltage clamp the membrane

In Stimulus Control, select VClamp. By default, you will deliver a 4 ms step from –65 mV to 0 mV. To look in detail at the rising phases and peaks of the currents, set the Total # (ms) to 4. (The clamp step will terminate off the graph.)

## 2. In the Kinetic Parameters Control panel, shift the gating of INa (m) 20 mV in both directions in 1 mV steps

If you Keep Lines, you can easily observe the <u>changes</u> in INa as you shift the activation relation. When shifted in the depolarizing direction, a greater depolarization is required to gate a given fraction of the channels. Return vshift_m (mV) to 0 and erase your traces.

## 3. Shift the inactivation curve for INa (h) 20 mV in both directions in a series of steps

There should be an obvious difference between the family of currents you observe in this experiment and those in the previous experiment where you shifted *m*.

## 4. Shift the gating of IK (n) 20 mV in both directions in 1 mV steps

In order to see the peak IK you should give a longer clamp Testing Level pulse, 15 ms, and set the Total # (ms) to 15.

Your observations on the gating relation for IK should be qualitatively similar to those for INa. That is, if the curve is shifted 20 mV to the left, there will be a finite IK at –100 mV and a steeply rising current of large amplitude. If it is shifted 20 mV to the right, IK will rise slowly and peak at a lower amplitude.

## OBSERVE *m* AND *h* DURING THE ACTION POTENTIAL

In the experiments below, we focus on the two determinants of the Na current and excitability, *m* and *h*. If you *really* hunger to see *n* as well, you can launch the *m-h-and-n-vs*-Time graph from the P&G Manager.

## 1. Observe m and h during an action potential evoked by depolarization

- **Launch the *m-and-h-vs*-Time graph.**
  Restore the default Total # (ms) (10 ms) by clicking the red square. Run the simulation to see the *m* and *h* values at the resting potential and then how *m* and *h* change during the action potential.

- **Relate the plot of *m* during the action potential to the *m* curve in the Kinetic Parameters Control graph.**
  Why does *m* surge to a value of 1—that is, to a probability that all of the Na channels are activated—and then linger for so long at that value, even as the action potential is in its falling phase? Measure the time at which *m* begins a rapid decrease. Where is the voltage at this time? By looking at the *m* curve in the Kinetic Parameters Control graph, can you <u>explain this relation</u> between *m* and the action potential?

- **Relate the plot of *h* during the action potential to the *h* curve in the Kinetic Parameters Control graph.**

  - Does it surprise you that *h* is at such a high value (0.6) at the resting potential? This means that only 60 percent of the Na channels are not inactivated and are available for opening at the resting potential. You can measure this value from the *h* curve in the Kinetic Parameters Control panel.

  - Because 40 percent of the channels are inactivated at rest, you will see, below, how making Vm more negative, through inhibition, can remove this inactivation and increase excitability.

  - Explain the behavior of *h* during the action potential. When is the *h* trace at a minimum (meaning the fewest channels available for opening)? <u>Why</u> does the *h* trace begin to recover its resting value even though the action potential bottoms at –76 mV, the trough of the undershoot?

## 2. *Observe m and h during an "<u>anode break</u>" action potential evoked at the offset of a hyperpolarizing current pulse*

Here, you can see how removing inactivation, by delivering a hyperpolarizing stimulus, gives neurons a whole new way to generate an action potential, leading to new possibilities for circuitry. This type of event, sometimes termed an "off response" or "disinhibition," is explored in more detail in the <u>Postsynaptic Inhibition</u> tutorial.

- **In IClamp, set the pulse parameters as follows:**

  - Set the delay to 0.5 ms.

  - Set the duration to 10 ms and the Total # (ms) to 30.

  - Set the amplitude, initially, to –0.03 nA.

- **Explain, in terms of *m* and *h*, <u>why</u> an anode-break action potential occurs.**
  Keep Lines and give additional current steps of –0.02 and –0.01 nA. Compare the *m* traces, *h* traces, and the action potentials in response to each stimulus. The same duration pulse leads to a very different delay in the action potential initiation, depending on pulse amplitude. The reason for this should be clear from inspection of the *m* and *h* curves. Since timing is crucial in neuronal integration, it is valuable to understand why this delay is so different for different degrees of "inhibition."

### SIMULATE DIFFERENT Na CHANNEL SUBTYPES

The Na channel family members display a range of *m* and *h* relations. Here, you can simulate how the different Na channel subtypes might affect membrane excitability.

This exercise should give you an appreciation for the functional variety of the Na channels. However, it cannot truly reproduce reality. In your simulations, the Na current through each channel subtype is competing with only the HH K current; whereas in real neurons, K channels come in a myriad of subtypes.

Further, there may be more than one subtype of Na channel present in a neuron. Nevertheless, the simulations may give you insight as to why there are channel subtypes by showing how they can affect neuronal excitability over a wide range.

## 1. Simulate a subtype

In this link, we have chosen values for $m$ and $h$ for each of the nine mammalian subtypes of Na channel based on averaged data from Catterall et al. (2003).

- **Choose a member of the family.**
  Go to the page of subtype kinetics values, linked above. Choose a subtype, and type the values of $m$ and $h$ for that subtype into their respective fields in your Kinetic Parameters Control window.

- **Run the simulation.**
  How would the particular Na channel subtype you have chosen affect excitability if it were in a membrane with the HH K channels? Repeating this exercise with other subtypes should give you a sense of the range over which the Na channels affect excitability.

## MIMIC THE ACTION OF TOXINS THAT AFFECT THE Na CHANNEL

The experiments here focus on four Na channel toxins: (1) Tetrodotoxin (TTX) from the puffer fish and certain salamanders, (2) maculotoxin from the blue-ringed octopus of Australia, (3) brevetoxin from the red tide of the Gulf of Mexico, and (4) batrachotoxin (BTX) from the skin of South American frogs.

## 1. Mimic the effects of TTX

You will be familiar with TTX if you have done the Na Action Potential tutorial. TTX, and a related molecule, saxitoxin (STX), from the red tide in New England waters, is a highly specific blocker of many (but not all) of the voltage-gated Na channel subtypes, including the HH Na channel. TTX and STX do not affect channel kinetics but only the amplitude of the Na current.

- **Voltage-clamp the membrane.**
  Record the normal Na current. Use the default parameters in VClamp and reset the Total # (ms) to 4.

- **Block the Na channels by reducing the Na channel density.**
  Decrease the Na channel density in the Patch Parameters panel. We suggest dividing the density value by two several times, and choosing Keep Lines so that you can examine the family. Notice that the rate of rise is halved with each division and that the peak currents occur at about the same time. Does TTX affect inactivation?

## 2. Mimic the effects of maculotoxin

Maculotoxin is a component of the saliva of the beautiful but extremely dangerous blue-ringed octopus. The beak of this golfball-sized animal is reported to be able to penetrate a wet suit; its bite will kill a person within minutes. Maculotoxin contains TTX as well as a second component that shifts the kinetics of the HH Na channel.

The figure shown here is taken from a study of the effect of maculotoxin on INa in a voltage-clamped squid axon. The different traces show the diminishing amplitude of the Na current as the toxin washes onto the preparation. Although maculotoxin contains TTX, this figure should look different from your observations with pure TTX (above). Use the simulation tools in this tutorial to discover for yourself what the second component is doing to the Na channel.

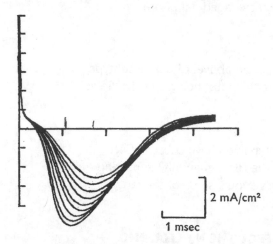

**2 mA/cm²**

**1 msec**

### 3. *Mimic the effects of brevetoxin*

Brevetoxin is produced by the red-tide organism, *Gymnodinium breve*. Rather than blocking Na channels, this toxin activates them, causing spontaneous, sustained firing of impulses that exhaust a nerve's energy supply.

Brevetoxin has two main actions on the Na channels of rat sensory neurons: (1) It shifts $m$ to more negative potentials, and (2) it inhibits inactivation of the Na channels. Westerfield et al. (1977), first reporting the action of brevetoxin by testing it on squid axon, marveled at "the dramatic change in the normal activity of the axon." What do you expect this "dramatic change" to be?

- **In the Kinetic Parameters Control panel, shift *m* by –10 mV to mimic the effects of brevetoxin.**
  Set the amplitude of the current pulse to zero and the Total # (ms) to 30 so that you can watch for spontaneous activity. It is useful to bring the $m$-and-$h$-vs-Time graph back up to watch $m$ as you shift its relation. Do you think this shift in $m$ is overkill, as it were, for killing prey?

- **Leaving *m* shifted, now shift *h* in a direction that removes inactivation.**
  It must be very clear through these simulations why this toxin is so dangerous.

### 4. *Mimic the effects of batrachotoxin* BTX

BTX has several effects on voltage-gated Na channels, all conspiring to open the channels unnaturally, depolarize neurons and muscle fibers, and kill the victim!

This figure from Bosmans et al. (2004), shows the effect of BTX on the voltage-gated Na channel subtype 1.8, a channel gaining importance in nociception. The square symbols show the *m* and *h* curves for this subtype before the application of the BTX. Application of the toxin (circles, 5 μm; triangles, 10 μm) shifted the *m* relation to the left and essentially blocked inactivation, shifting the *h* relation upwards.

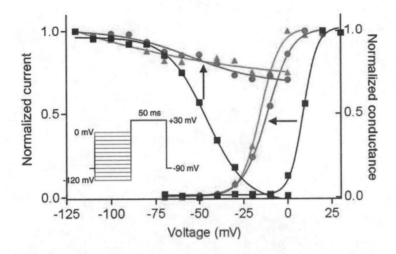

By simulating these changes in *m* and *h*, you can see the effects of BTX on the action potential.

- **In the Kinetic Parameters Control panel, select values of *m* and *h* for this subtype before BTX application.**
  Choose values that give curves that are as close as possible to those in the figure above. A more detailed description of the figure is provided <u>here</u>.

- **Now select values of *m* and *h* that approximate the curves after BTX application.**
  You should be able to simulate the *m* curve rather well. You cannot change the basic shape of the *h* curve in the simulation in order to mimic the incomplete block of inactivation seen in the figure, so you will have to block inactivation completely over the range tested (by moving the *h* curve far to the right).

- **What is the effect of BTX on the action potential?**
  You may have to increase the amplitude of the stimulus pulse to elicit an action potential. What do you think is the more effective action of this toxin in disrupting normal excitable membrane function—the blocking of inactivation or the shifting of the activation curve, *m*, to more negative voltages?

Keep in mind that the HH K channel is not blocked by this toxin and can repolarize the membrane. Is there a degree of shift of the *m* curve that gives such a large advantage to the Na current over the K current that the action potential won't repolarize?

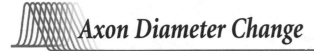

## How Does an Axon's Impulse Invade a Soma?

**How does an action potential travel in a neuron with complicated geometry?**
What happens to the action potential when it encounters a branch point or
when it tries to invade a cell body? This tutorial explores the transmission of
impulses through a region of a neuron where there is an abrupt change in
diameter (in the default example, a tenfold change). You are recording from
the cell in five locations: three locations in the smaller axon and two locations
in the larger axon (see diagram).

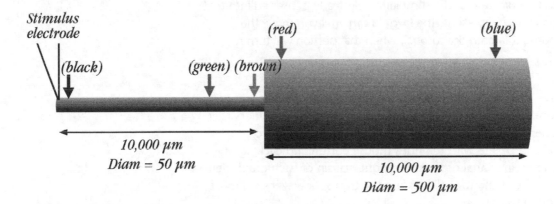

**You will experiment with an unmyelinated axon's diameter change.**
The smaller-diameter (50 μm) segment on the left may be thought of as a
branch of the larger-diameter (500 μm) axon on the right. Indeed, the 500
μm-diameter squid giant axon often has 50 μm-diameter branches. You can
specify the diameters of these segments. The inhomogeneous axon in this
tutorial may also be thought of as an axon and cell soma.

### Goals of this Tutorial
• To observe impulses in the smaller axon struggling to invade the larger axon
  and understand the curious current patterns that result from the struggle
• To explore how the ratio of the two diameters affects the ability of the action
  potential to invade the larger-diameter axon
• To experiment with how temperature changes affect invasion of the larger-
  diameter axon
• To understand why impulses move with no difficulty from the larger to the
  smaller axon

## Start the Simulation

Click this button to bring up the panels and windows of the simulation.

    Start the Simulation

## Description of the Panels and Windows Customized for this Tutorial

### 1. Assumptions

This tutorial assumes that you are completely familiar with the manipulations of the *NIA* tutorials. A familiarity with the Partial Demyelination tutorial would also be helpful.

### 2. The stimulating electrode

The stimulating electrode is at the left end (0) of the small axon (red portion of line). The line is red to indicate that the stimulating electrode is inserted into that component. The **black line** represents the **large axon** until you move the electrode to this segment later in the tutorial, when that portion will turn red.

### 3. The graphs

- **The Voltage-vs-Time and Na Current-vs-Time graphs:** With five recording sites (color-coded as in the diagram above), you will have to work harder than usual to keep track of all of the traces. Remember that you can delete traces by choosing Delete with the right mouse button and clicking on their labels, shown in spatial order at the right margin of each graph (left-most recording site at the top). To restore the traces, however, you must close and re-open the graph.

- **The Voltage-vs-Space graph:** The sites of the recording electrodes are indicated by arrowheads along the *x*-axis.

## Experiments and Observations

### OBSERVE PROPAGATION FROM A SMALLER DIAMETER PROCESS INTO A LARGER DIAMETER REGION

### 1. Observe the impulse in the Voltage-vs-Space window

Run the simulation. There is much to observe as the impulse, initiated at the left end of the smaller axon, moves into the large-diameter axon and then is initiated again in the smaller axon:

- The change in shape of the rising phase of the advancing impulse when it encounters the junction between the two segments

- The voltage profile in the large axon as the voltage hesitates at threshold

- The voltage profile as it finally gives an action potential in the large axon

- The changing amplitude of the action potential at the junction as it re-establishes itself in the small-diameter axon

To understand these changes, it will be useful to look at the graphs of voltage and current versus time.

### 2. *Study the traces in the Voltage-vs-Time graph*

It is probably most useful to run the simulation over and over, and watch each trace as the action potential moves from left to right and then bounces back from right to left. The black electrode will record the voltage first—and last. Relate the Voltage-vs-Time recordings at a selected electrode to the impulse moving past that electrode in the Voltage-vs-Space graph.

- Question: Is it clear from the movie why the second green action potential has a smaller amplitude than the first?

- Question: Is it clear why the red recording electrode begins to record a depolarization before the blue electrode but then records the action potential later than the blue electrode?

### 3. *Study the Na currents*

You should by now recognize and understand the "kinky" shape of the Na current.

- Question: What is the most eye-catching current in this group of Na current recordings?

- Question: Why is the the Na current larger near the junction?

## HOW DOES PROPAGATION FROM THE SMALLER INTO THE LARGER AXON DEPEND ON THE RATIO OF THE DIAMETERS?

### 1. *Bring up the Small Axon Parameters panel*

Experiment with diameter to see how the diameter of the small axon affects the ability of the impulse to propagate into the large axon. You may want to delete all of the current traces except the interesting ones (brown and red) at the junction, and then use Keep Lines to compare simulations at different diameters.

(Remember that you delete traces by choosing Delete with the right mouse button and clicking on the label; you restore them by closing and re-opening the graph.)

### 2. *Reduce the diameter*

The default diameter ratio was set near the critical value. By how much must you reduce the small axon's diameter in order to cause failure of invasion of the large axon?

### 3. *Increase the diameter*

What magnitude of increase will speed propagation into the large axon? Will merely a small increase in the diameter of the small axon be sufficient, or must the diameters of the two processes be much closer in size to one another?

### 4. *Experiment with other variables*

We have left other parameters in the Small Axon Parameters menu for you to change if you wish. A menu for changing parameters in the large-diameter axon may also be called up. What happens to propagation if you change the capacitance of either of these segments? What happens if you change a channel density? Using impulse invasion as an assay, you can thoroughly test your knowledge of neurophysiology!

## INVESTIGATE HOW INVASION DEPENDS ON TEMPERATURE

### 1. *Restore the default parameters*

Reset the diameter of the small axon to the default value of 50 µm.

### 2. *Think, then change the temperature*

Will cooling or warming improve transmission from the smaller to the larger axon? Recall your experiments with temperature in the Na Action Potential and the Partial Demyelination tutorials. Will the same principles in those tutorials apply to the present experiment? A discussion of the effects of temperature on the impulse and its propagation is available.

### 3. *Study the voltage change and the Na current at the junction*

If you have not done so by now, delete all of the traces in the Voltage-vs-Time and the Current-vs-Time plots except for the brown traces recorded in the small-diameter axon at the junction. Use Keep Lines to compare the recordings at several temperatures. How sharp is the temperature dependence of impulse invasion?

## REVERSE THE DIRECTION OF PROPAGATION

### 1. *Relaunch the Voltage-vs-Time and the Current-vs-Time graphs so that all of the traces can re-appear*

### 2. *Move the electrode to the far-right end of the large axon*

If you now run the simulation, you will find that there is insufficient default-stimulus current to generate a spike in the large axon. Why?

### 3. *Increase the stimulus current amplitude tenfold*

You will see that the impulse is generated and travels smoothly from right to left with no hesitation; the only noticeable change is that the wavelength of the spike (or spatial extent) becomes shorter in the small-diameter region. (Why is this the case?) The Na current density is almost constant in all locations. In other words, in this direction, the impulse traverses the diameter change with ease. If you have worked through the exercises of this tutorial, you should completely understand this observation.

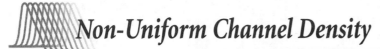

## Altering Impulse Conduction with Local Anesthetics

**What happens when conduction is blocked locally with an anesthetic?**
Can an action potential propagate through a region whose channels are blocked by anesthetics or toxins? In this tutorial, you will explore how a change in the density of functioning channels affects impulse propagation through the region containing those channels.

**The preparation**
In this tutorial we look at three squid axon segments, each 10,000 μm (10 mm) long. Records of the membrane potential are taken in the center of each of the segments, as indicated by the arrows on the diagram. Remember that NEURON views channel density and conductance as equivalent: Blocking a fraction of the channels, for example with an anesthetic, is the same as decreasing the density of functioning channels, as shown in the middle section of the diagram.

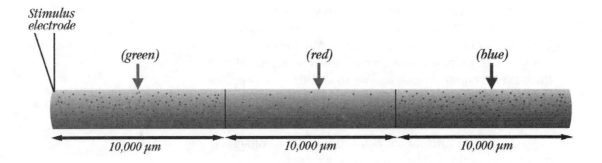

**Goals of this Tutorial**
- To test how local application of tetrodotoxin, a Na channel blocker, affects propagation
- To test how local application of 4-aminopyridine (4AP), a K channel blocker, affects propagation
- To test how application of the anesthetic lidocaine, which affects both conductances, alters impulse propagation through the anesthetized region
- To test how local trauma affects propagation

## Start the Simulation

Click this button to bring up the panels and windows of the simulation.

    Start the Simulation

## Description of the Panels and Windows Customized for this Tutorial

### 1. Assumptions

This tutorial assumes that you are familiar with all of the manipulations of the *NIA* tutorials.

### 2. The stimulating electrode

The Stimulus Control panel shows that the electrode is located at the left end of the axon. The leftmost third of the line is red, indicating that this is the segment under control of the stimulus. Check the pulse parameters: You will be stimulating with a short, sharp shock.

### 3. The graphs

- **The Voltage-vs-Time and Na Current-vs-Time graphs:** The color-coded labels of the three recording electrodes are stacked in spatial order, with the leftmost electrode at the top. Run the simulation to see the three recordings of the action potential. Your trained neurophysiological eye will probably notice immediately that the peak amplitude of the action potential increases and the peak Na current decreases ever so slightly as the impulse travels from left to right (you can check this with the crosshairs). This results from the way the tutorial was set up. Can you guess why?

- **The Voltage-vs-Space graph:** Arrowheads color-coded to the Voltage-vs-Time traces indicate the position of the recording electrodes.

## Experiments and Observations

### BLOCK Na CHANNELS WITH TETRODOTOXIN (TTX) IN THE MIDDLE SEGMENT

### 1. Apply a toxin highly specific for Na channels only in the middle portion of the axon

Bring up the Middle Axon Parameters menu. Use tetrodotoxin (TTX), a very powerful toxin made by the puffer fish (about 1 mg is a lethal dose for a person). Reduce the maximum Na channel density (Na conductance) several-fold in the middle axon segment.

### 2. How much block can the axon tolerate?

Observe carefully the voltage patterns as the impulse in the middle segment begins to fail. Find out by how much you can block Na conductance and still be able to recover an impulse in the right axon segment. Use Keep Lines to compare voltage and current traces as you gradually block Na conductance.

You may have found a particular value for the Na conductance that caused a reflection from the right segment back into the middle segment. Why does this occur? Hint: Note the timing of the action potential in the rightmost segment under normal and blocked conditions.

### 3. *Restore default values*

Remember to restore the default value of the conductance(s) after this and each of the following experiments.

## BLOCK K CHANNELS WITH AN AMINOPYRIDINE

### 1. *Apply a K channel blocker to the middle segment*

Apply 4AP, a blocker specific for the HH K channel, by reducing the K conductance in the middle section. Interpret your observations.

## BLOCK BOTH Na AND K CHANNELS WITH LOCAL ANESTHETICS

### 1. *Apply lidocaine to the middle segment*

Anesthetics such as procaine and lidocaine affect both the Na and the K conductances about equally. Reduce both the Na and the K conductances twofold, fivefold, and tenfold. Guess what will happen before running the simulation in each case: The result may not be as straightforward as you think it will be.

- Question: Can you explain why the impulse is delayed in propagating into the right-hand section?

### 2. *Compare blocking both conductances simultaneously with blocking them separately*

- Question: Can you explain the different effects of TTX and lidocaine on the impulse in the central section?

## INVESTIGATE THE EFFECTS OF TRAUMA

Mechanical trauma can damage nerve membranes and their proteins, making them more leaky to ions and overwhelming the pumps that maintain the intracellular Na concentration at a low value and K concentration at a high value.

### 1. *Damage the middle segment*

Simulate an increased leakiness by increasing the leakage conductance twofold, fivefold, tenfold, and 50-fold. The leakiness will cause the middle segment to depolarize. By how much can you increase the leakage conductance and still maintain transmission to the right segment?

This experiment should give you an idea of how much damage an axon impaled with a sharp microelectrode can sustain if the electrode causes damage in the process of insertion.

### 2. *Block the Na pump in the middle segment*

Simulate damage to the Na pump in the middle segment by reducing ENa by, for example, 5, 10, 20, and 50 mV. When does transmission fail?

### *3. How much length can be damaged before transmission fails*

With ENa reduced, increase the length of the middle segment. When you do this, the left segment will be forced off the graph to the left on the Voltage-vs-Space plot and you will have to wait for the action potential to arrive on the plot after the stimulus pulse is given. If you have made the middle segment very long, you will have to increase the time of running the simulation in the "Total (#) ms" field. Are you surprised to learn how much local damage a nerve can tolerate?

The View = plot option will allow you to see the entire length of the axon, but the labels for the recording electrodes will no longer be at the correct locations.

## PLAY WITH *NIA*

### *1. Change parameters of the end segments*

Click on the "Left & Right Axon Parameters" button to bring up panels in which to change the values of parameters in these segments. They afford the possibility of exploring a large variety of interactions.

### *2. Change the temperature*

Investigate the effect of a temperature change, combined with local changes in conductance. Your experience, gained in earlier tutorials, ought to allow you to predict the outcome of such experiments.

## CONCLUSIONS

This tutorial reveals that there is a lot of resilience built into the impulse-generating mechanism. A large "safety factor" ensures transmission in the face of considerable difficulties. Whenever the struggling impulse in the middle segment manages to bring the right segment to threshold, the action potential there quickly resumes its normal shape and continues on.

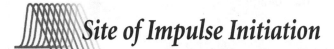

# Site of Impulse Initiation

## How Geometry Affects Where the Impulse Initiates

**Where in the intact neuron does the action potential initiate?**
Is it triggered in the dendrites, in the soma, in the "initial segment" of the axon, or further out in the axon itself? That this question has inspired many <u>experimental approaches</u> since Jack Eccles first asked it in the 1950s speaks to its importance for our understanding of how neurons integrate information. This first tutorial in the Cells section of *NIA* allows you to experiment with changes in neuronal geometry and observe how they affect the site of impulse initiation.

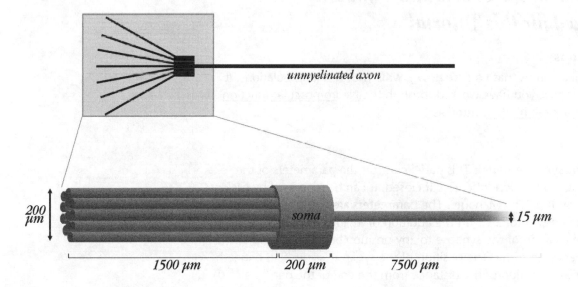

**The neuron in this tutorial is "stylized," meaning it is the simplest computational representation of a neuron.**
In the following experiments you will simulate voltage changes in a neuron with the simplest possible morphology, comprising the following regions (from left to right on the diagram):

- A single, passive dendrite representing the entire dendritic arbor of the neuron, <u>collapsed</u> into a cylinder as shown in the diagram, contacted by a single synapse; the position of the synapse along the dendrite may be adjusted
- A soma with voltage-gated HH Na and K channels
- An *unmyelinated* axon with HH Na and K channels

**Goals of this Tutorial**
- To interpret movies of impulse initiation and voltage distribution along the cell in response to synaptic input onto its dendrite

- To experiment with the effects of the following parameters on the voltage distribution:
  - The strength of the synaptic input on the dendrite
  - The location of the synapse on the dendrite
  - Changes in the diameter or length of the soma
  - Changes in the diameter of the axon
  - Changes in ion channel densities

## Start the Simulation

Click this button to bring up the panels and windows of the simulation.

**Start the Simulation**

## Description of the Panels and Windows Customized for this Tutorial

### 1. Assumptions

This tutorial assumes that you are now a whiz with *NIA* manipulations. It also assumes that you have worked through the Neuromuscular Junction and Postsynaptic Inhibition tutorials.

### 2. The panels

- **The AlphaSynapse panel:** This panel controls the parameters of the single input to the dendritic tree. If closed, it can be reopened by clicking a button on the P&G Manager. The parameters are the same as in similar panels in earlier tutorials with the addition of a slider that allows you to move the location of the synapse to any position between the tip of the dendrite and the soma. The position of the synapse is specified beneath the slider as a fraction of the distance from the end of the dendrite (1.0) to the soma (0.0).

- **The Cell Parameters panel:** This panel allows you to control the parameters in each segment of the cell separately. The titles of each section of the panel point out that the dendrites are passive (no voltage-gated channels), while the soma and axon are active (HH Na and K channels).

### 3. The graphs

- **The Voltage-vs-Time plot (upper right):**

  - The recording electrode in the dendrite is located in the middle, or 0.5, position; because of its length, the dendrite will not be isopotential.

  - The soma, on the other hand, is isopotential; the recording electrode is located in the 0.5 position, but the precise location does not really matter because of the isopotentiality.

  - The recording electrode in the axon is located at the 0.1 position, one-tenth of the distance from the soma to the axon's end.

- **The Voltage-vs-Space plot (lower right):** The dimensions of the dendritic tree, soma, and axon comprising the *x*-axis are shown on the diagram above. The positions of the three recording electrodes are indicated on the *x*-axis by the color-coded arrowheads.

## Experiments and Observations

### WHERE IS THE SITE OF SPIKE INITIATION?

### 1. *Deliver a suprathreshold EPSP to the middle of the dendrite*

Note the default parameters in the AlphaSynapse panel, then click R&R. By studying the movie in the steps suggested below, observe where the impulse initiates when the synapse is at its default location in the middle of the dendrite.

### 2. *Study the movie and Voltage-vs-Time traces*

Using Reset, then "Continue for (ms)" in steps of 0.2 ms, look carefully at the sequence of voltage changes in each domain of the neuron. Also look at each of the three recordings in the Voltage-vs-Time plot.

- Question: Can you discern precisely where the impulse initiates and why?

- Question: Why is the action potential in the soma of reduced amplitude compared to that in the axon? Is this voltage change an action potential?

- Question: Why does the dendrite appear to give an action potential (or at least a voltage change similar to that in the soma) when it has been specified to contain no voltage-sensitive ion channels?

### CAN THE SITE OF IMPULSE INITIATION BE ALTERED BY PARAMETER CHANGES?

Could the default settings have been selected to cause initiation in the axon? Was this a setup?

### 1. *Change the synaptic strength (conductance)*

- Double, then redouble the synaptic conductance (gmax).

- Question: Has the site of initiation changed with synaptic strength?

### 2. *Change the location of the synapse on the dendrite*

- Return the synaptic conductance setting to its default value.

- In the AlphaSynapse Manager, move the synapse first to the distal and then to the proximal end of the dendrite and run the simulation in each location.

- Question: Has the site of initiation changed with synaptic location?

### 3. *Change the diameter and length of the soma*

- Return the synapse to its default location.

- In the Active Soma Parameters section of the Cell Parameters panel, make the following changes and run the simulations:

- Change the soma's diameter to one-half, then to four times its default value of 200 μm.

- Double and halve the soma's length from its default value of 200 μm.

• Question: Can you <u>explain your results</u> when you change the soma morphology?

## 4. *Change the diameter of the axon*

• In the Soma Parameters section, restore the soma's diameter and length to their default values of 200 μm each.

• In the Active Axon Parameters section:

- Change the axon's diameter to one-half, then to four times its default value of 15 μm.

- As you increase the axon's diameter, you may want to increase the synaptic strength (gmax) to keep the time of spike generation approximately the same.

• Question: Has the site of initiation or the relative timing of the spike in the soma and axon <u>changed</u> with axon diameter?

## 5. *Change the ion channel densities*

In freeze-fracture electron micrographs of axons taken at high power, there appears to be an increase in the number of particles in the membrane of the initial segment of axons relative to other regions. There is now experimental evidence that these particles may be channels. You can explore the effect of changes in axonal channel densities in the next experiments.

• Restore (if altered) the synaptic strength to its default value.

• In the Active Axon Parameters section:

- Restore the axon's diameter to its default value of 15 μm.

- Run the simulation and use Keep Lines in the Voltage-vs-Time window.

- Halve, then double the densities of both the Na and K channels.

- Leave the Na channel density doubled but return the K channel density to its default value to see the effect of doubling the Na channel density alone.

• Question: Have changes in ion channel densities <u>affected</u> the site of impulse initiation or the relative timing of the spike in the soma and axon?

## SUMMARY

A neuron's morphology *per se* causes the spike to initiate in the axon in a region close to the soma. The probability that this region is the site of initiation can be increased by an increased density of Na channels at this location. Mounting evidence suggests that the initial segments of axons of some neurons have just such an extra dose of Na channels.

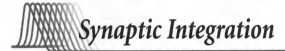

# Synaptic Integration

## Explore Integration of Excitatory and Inhibitory Inputs on Multiple Dendrites

**In this tutorial you will simulate a simplified spinal motoneuron of the cat.**
NEURON is capable of handling the full set of descriptive details of a real neuron: its morphology (measured from dye-labeled cells), channel types, channel locations and densities, and synaptic locations throughout the full dendritic tree. In this tutorial, we will restrict these parameters to a <u>manageable subset</u>.

**A simplified neuron can be surprisingly complex.**
Even with the reduced parameter set available in this tutorial, you may begin to feel overwhelmed by the complexity introduced by the limited set of possibilities here. There is much to be learned simply by changing the strengths, locations, reversal potentials, and onset times of the three synaptic inputs on the dendrites. We hope this tutorial will raise your sensitivity to oversimplifications in interpretation of published observations.

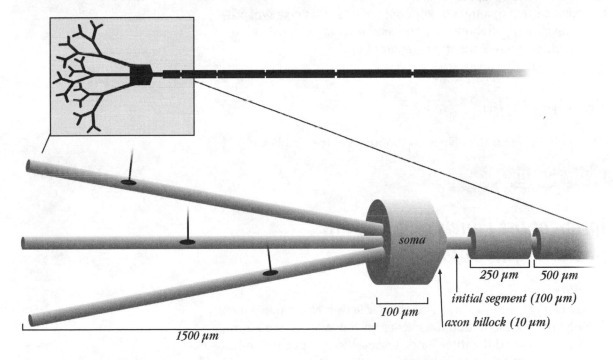

**This "stylized" motoneuron has five different sections.**
- **The dendritic tree:** The dendritic tree is now represented by three dendrites 1.5 mm in length and 24 μm in diameter, each with synaptic inputs whose location, strength, and timing may be controlled.
- **The soma:** The soma is represented by a cylinder 100 μm by 100 μm.
- **The axon hillock:** The axon hillock is the 10 μm region where the soma tapers from 100 μm to the 10 μm diameter of the specialized region called the "initial segment" of the axon.

- **The initial segment:** Between the axon hillock and the axon is the initial segment of the axon, 100 μm in length and 10 μm in diameter, where the axon is bare—not yet myelinated.
- **The axon:** The rest of the axon, 12 mm (12000 μm) in length, is myelinated (rather than bare, as in the Site of Impulse Initiation tutorial). You will explore whether the presence of myelin is important in determining the site of impulse initiation.

**The densities of the channels in the various segments have been chosen based on experimental evidence.**
The channel densities in each structural component have been chosen to match available experimental observations in the spinal motoneuron of the cat. For didactic purposes, the dendrites in this tutorial are passive, although it is now known that the dendrites of CNS neurons can have voltage-gated channels in their membranes.

**Goals of this Tutorial**
- To compare the site of impulse initiation in this neuron, whose axon is myelinated, with that in the unmyelinated axon in the Site of Impulse Initiation tutorial
- To explore how impulse initiation depends on each of the following:
  - The timing of the synaptic inputs on each of three dendrites
  - The location of these synapses
  - The temporal pattern in a train of impulses arriving at a single synapse
  - The temporal pattern, strength, location, and reversal potential of the synaptic inputs on each of the three dendrites

## Start the Simulation

Click this button to bring up the panels and windows of the simulation.

> **Start the Simulation**

## Description of the Panels and Windows Customized for this Tutorial

### 1. Assumptions

This tutorial assumes that you are incredibly facile with *NIA* manipulations, even making right-mouse-button discoveries on your own. It also assumes that you have completed the three Patch tutorials on synaptic transmission in the Basic section and the Site of Impulse Initiation tutorial.

### 2. The AlphaSynapse panels

Each of the experiments in this tutorial has a special, dedicated AlphaSynapse panel that permits you to change certain variables of the synapse. Each of these panels will appear in the same position (lower-left portion of the monitor) when you launch it from its button in the P&G Manager. When you click Start the Simulation, the AlphaSynapse panel for the first experiment, entitled "Vary Onsets and Locations" (see also, title in bar at the top of the panel), comes up automatically.

The "Vary Onsets and Locations" AlphaSynapse panel allows you to change certain variables of the synapses on the three dendrites:

- **The conductance**, which in this menu is the same for all inputs

- **The onset** of each synaptic potential, which can be adjusted for each synapse separately

- **The location** of each synapse on the dendrite, adjustable by a slider for each synapse as shown in the diagram

The text line just below the three sliders shows, from left to right, the location of each synapse as a fraction of the distance from the end (1) of the dendrite to the soma (0).

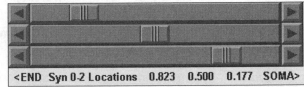

<END  Syn 0-2 Locations   0.823   0.500   0.177   SOMA>

### 3. The graphs

- **The Voltage-vs-Time plot (upper right):** Four electrodes record the voltage change in the soma and axon in these color-coded positions:

  - In the soma (thicker trace, brown)

  - At node [0] (0.35 mm from soma, red)

  - At node [1] (1.1 mm from soma, blue)

  - At node [5] (5.1 mm from soma, black)

- **The Voltage-vs-Space plot (lower right):** The dimensions of the dendritic tree, soma, and 5-mm-long portion of the axon comprising this *x*-axis are shown on the diagram above. The positions of the four recording electrodes are indicated on the axis by the color-coded arrowheads.

- **The Extend-Voltage-vs-Space plot (launched from P&G Manager):** This graph extends the *x*-axis from 5000 μm to 12000 μm, which allows you to see where the impulse initiates in the axon.

## Experiments and Observations

### GENERATE EPSPS IN THE DENDRITES
### AND OBSERVE WHERE THE SPIKE INITIATES

### 1. Press R&R to deliver three EPSPs 0.5 ms apart at three dendritic locations

In this first simulation, note the staggered locations of the inputs (EPSPs) to the three dendrites by checking the positions on the sliders. They occur in sequence—at 0 ms for the input onto the black dendrite, 0.5 ms for the input onto the red dendrite, and 1 ms for the input onto the blue dendrite.

### 2. Find where the spike is initiated

The Voltage-vs-Space plot shows only the initial 5000 μm of axon. Launch the Extend-Voltage-vs-Space plot to see the full 12000 μm length of this myelinated axon. Now, examine both plots to see if you can determine where the spike is initiated.

### 3. *Examine the voltage change in the initial segment and axon*

For a paused-action view of the sequence of events, advance the movie with the "Reset" and "Continue for (ms)" buttons in increments of 0.1 ms or another value of your choice. Notice especially the voltage change in the initial segment. Why is it so steep?

### 4. *Examine the voltage change in the soma and dendrites*

The impulse, initiated in the axon, backpropagates into the soma, its peak amplitude progressively decreasing from node[5] to node[0]. The soma struggles, unable to depolarize even up to 0 mV. Backpropagation of the depolarization continues into the dendritic tree, where most of each dendrite is depolarized to about –40 mV.

- Question: Recent experiments reveal that action potentials can back-propagate into the dendritic tree in certain CNS neurons. What effect would this dendritic depolarization have on subsequent synaptic inputs on a dendrite? Click here for a discussion of this question.

### 5. *Reverse the timing or locations of the EPSPs so that the EPSP near the soma comes first*

Deliver the first EPSP near the soma and the last near a dendritic end. You can do this either (1) by simply reversing the values of the onset times for Syn 0 Black and Syn 2 Blue, leaving their locations the same, or (2) by reversing synapse locations, as shown below. The EPSP occurring first will now be closest to the cell soma. Will this sequence of EPSPs cause an action potential to initiate? Click here for a discussion of this experiment. Try moving the location of the most distal synapse to see how its position affects your results.

Original locations:

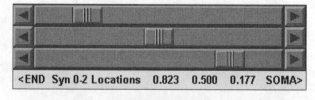

Reversed locations:

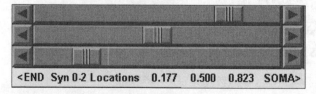

## DELIVER A TRAIN OF SYNAPTIC INPUTS AT A SINGLE SYNAPTIC LOCATION

The temporal pattern of impulses in a train arriving at a synapse is thought to be important in determining whether or not a neuron fires. In this tutorial you can arrange to have the three EPSPs arrive at one synapse on one dendrite, simulating the first three impulses of a train.

### 1. *Bring up a new AlphaSynapse menu*

Click the "Train, Single Location" button in the Panel Manager. There is no need to close the previous menu; the new one will replace it.

**Trains in NEURON**
The simulator views a train as three synapses at the same location (indicated by the slider position), in this case on the red dendrite. The onset of each EPSP is set independently.

## 2. *Deliver the train*

Run the simulation with the default parameters and watch the movie of the three EPSPs. The conductance increases have been made the same for each EPSP to keep this experiment from becoming too complex. Look carefully at the amplitudes of the EPSPs: With identical conductance increases, do they add linearly? If you have completed the Interactions of Postsynaptic Potentials tutorial, you should be able to explain how the EPSPs add.

## 3. *For bringing the neuron to threshold, are EPSPs in a train equivalent to those same EPSPs occurring simultaneously?*

When neurotransmitter (released from the presynaptic terminal) causes a conductance change in a dendrite, which gives rise to a synaptic current, that current flows forward in the cell to depolarize the region of spike initiation. The amount of current is the important factor in whether the neuron will depolarize enough to initiate an action potential. Will three EPSPs in a train cause less, more, or the same amount of current to enter the cell as three EPSPs occurring simultaneously?

- **Determine the threshold conductance for the three EPSPs in the train at the 0.5 location.**
  A fast way to search for the threshold conductance is to use the arrows in the spinner box to make your changes, because a simulation will automatically run when you make the change. (Reminder: Clicking the right mouse button on the UP arrow in the spinner box will allow you to select the decade in which the arrows of the box make changes.)

  Keep in mind, in thinking about the relevance of these experiments to CNS integration, that conductance is equivalent to the amount of neurotransmitter gating the postsynaptic receptors on the dendrites.

- **Now set all three onset times to 0 ms and determine the threshold conductance again.**
  Explain your results. As an advanced exercise to test your explanation, you can experiment with the timing of the EPSPs in the train. What is the lowest synaptic conductance at which you can produce an impulse by playing with the interspike intervals?

## 4. *How does threshold change for the EPSPs in the train, and for those occurring simultaneously, as a function of synapse position on the dendrite?*

Find the threshold synaptic conductance as a function of the position of the synapse along the dendrite for the EPSPs occurring in the train. What do these relations tell you about voltage spread in a passive dendritic arbor?

## HOW DOES INHIBITORY SYNAPTIC INPUT (AN IPSP) AT ONE SYNAPSE AFFECT VOLTAGE SPREAD AND IMPULSE INITIATION?

### 1. Press the "All Synaptic Variables" button

The AlphaSynapse menu that is called up allows you to vary four parameters for each synapse:

- Conductance

- Onset

- Location

- Reversal potential

### 2. Make one synaptic input an IPSP

Set the reversal potential of one of the synapses to a value more negative than the resting potential of –70 mV. Run the simulation. You have the tools to do a large number of experiments with this neuron. For example, you can test parameters that might change the effectiveness of the IPSP in blocking impulses generated by one or two EPSPs. (You can set a conductance to zero to remove an input.) For the IPSP, explore the effect of changing the following:

- Its onset time with respect to EPSPs

- Its location

- Its conductance change

- The value of its reversal potential

### 3. Not satisfied? Change the temperature

If you find these experiments insufficiently challenging, you can investigate how temperature affects spike generation for the whole parameter set!

# Impulse Invasion of the Presynaptic Terminal

## Using Simulations to Understand Experimental Observations

**How does an action potential in a myelinated axon invade the axon's unmyelinated presynaptic terminal?**
In the Synaptic Integration tutorial, the impulse, generated in the myelinated axon of a motoneuron, sets off at high speed toward its destination, the muscle fiber. After a few milliseconds, we pick it up at the end of its journey over the last few nodes as it flies into the axon's presynaptic terminal arborization. Here, it faces a challenge—a sudden increase in capacitance due to the increased, unmyelinated membrane area required to house the hundreds of sites of transmitter release. Are there design features that help it invade this arbor?

**Simulations of experimental observations can shed light on this question.**
This tutorial shows how simulations can advance understanding when the ability to gain that knowledge through experiments is limited. In this case, the experimenters recorded currents flowing into the presynaptic arbor at a neuromuscular junction (NMJ) and then used NEURON to predict a channel density distribution throughout the arbor that would cause simulations to match those currents as closely as possible. Thus, the simulations set up a new hypothesis, one of channel density distribution, that eventually could be tested by other experimental approaches.

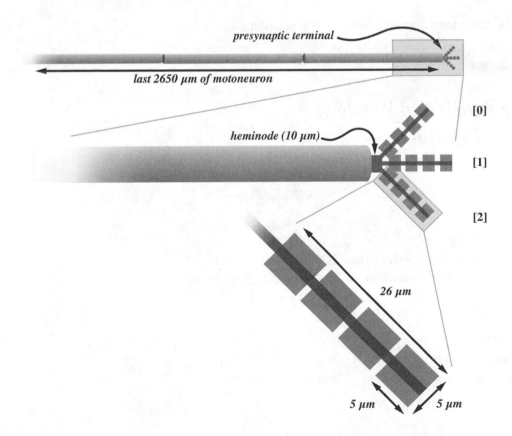

presynaptic terminal

last 2650 μm of motoneuron

[0]

heminode (10 μm)

[1]

[2]

26 μm

5 μm      5 μm

**This tutorial simulates experiments at the presynaptic terminal at a bouton-type NMJ.**

The bouton-type NMJ of the lizard was chosen for these experiments. In the simulation, this terminal has three main parts: (1) A myelinated axon; (2) a region called the "heminode," where the axon loses its myelin before arborizing; and (3) the presynaptic arbor, modeled as three branches, each with four boutons. This stylized morphology is based on published light- and electron-microscopic observations.

**In this tutorial you will follow the path of matching simulation to experiment.** After observing the action potential at selected recording sites, you will observe the current patterns along the arbor, as was done experimentally. Then, you will see how the simulator can reconstruct these current patterns—by making iterative guesses about ion channel density distribution—and, thereby, predict the voltages in the heminode and the boutons of the presynaptic arbor.

**Goals of this Tutorial**

- To observe the action potential as recorded in the three major portions of the presynaptic terminal: in the myelinated axon, at the termination of the myelin (the heminode), and along one branch of the presynaptic arbor
- To compare simulated currents in the arbor with experimental observations
- To experiment with changes in arbor geometry and conductances, observing how they change the currents
- To observe how changes in channel density and internode length affect invasion of the arbor

## Start the Simulation

Click this button to bring up the panels and windows of the simulation.

> **Start the Simulation**

## Description of the Panels and Windows Customized for this Tutorial

### 1. Assumptions

This tutorial assumes that you have completed the Myelinated Axon and the Partial Demyelination tutorials.

### 2. The Panel & Graph Manager

Buttons call up Parameters panels for the three main sections of the axon's presynaptic terminal (axon, heminode, and boutons). The channel densities in these panels are based on the published model that will be explored in this tutorial.

### 3. The stimulating electrode

The Stimulus Control panel shows that the axon is stimulated at its far left end, node[3], to set up the action potential. You will not be asked to make changes in the stimulus location or settings, but the panel must be open in order to stimulate the axon.

**ATTENTION!** *Do not close the Stimulus Control panel. It must be open to stimulate the axon.*

### 4. The graphs

- **The Voltage-vs-Space graph:** This graph will display the voltage as a function of the length of the entire axon to the tip of its arbor comprising the 4000 μm myelinated portion, the 10 μm heminode, and the 28 μm middle branch of the arbor.

  - The axon comprises four 998 μm internodes interrupted by four nodes, each 2 μm in length. The stimulus is located in left-most node, at the start of the Voltage-vs-Space plot.

  - The unmyelinated heminode is 10 μm long.

  - Beginning 2 μm from the heminode, each terminal arbor branch consists of four boutons (5 μm in both diameter and length) connected by four tiny processes 2 μm long; thus, each branch is 28 μm in total length.

  - The branches are numbered by NEURON as branch[0], [1], and [2] from top to bottom, but we will always be concerned with the middle branch, [1].

- **The Voltage-vs-Space, Terminal graph:** This graph shows the final 50 μm of the axon and terminal arbor at greater spatial resolution, allowing you to see events in the arbor.

**ATTENTION!** *Resizing this graph may cause the trace to disappear.*

- **The Voltages-vs-Time graph:** The traces on this graph are color-coded to eight recording locations: at the four nodes of the axon; in the heminode; and in the first three boutons of the terminal branch, as described in the first experiment below.

- **The Terminal-Currents-vs-Time graph:** The traces in this graph are recorded by five electrodes, beginning in the heminode and then progressing outward through the four boutons of branch[1]. The position of each trace is color-coded and labeled on the graph.

## Experiments and Observations

### VIEW MOVIES OF AN IMPULSE PROPAGATING ALONG THE AXON AND INTO THE NERVE TERMINAL

### 1. View the action potential in the Voltage-vs-Space graph

When you run the simulation, the axon will be stimulated at its left end. Notice the cusps at the nodes that you observed previously in the <u>Myelinated Axon</u> tutorial. Also, notice that the amplitude of the impulse falls off as it approaches the arbor but that it grows again in the heminode, only to fall off steeply in the branch; that is, it looks like the impulse might be having trouble invading the arbor, but it recovers as it progresses.

## 2. *Focus on the terminal arbor*

Bring up the Voltage-vs-Space, Terminal Region graph. (It will partially overlay the Voltage-vs-Space graph.) This voltage trace includes a small portion of the end of the last internode, the heminode, and the terminal branch, as labeled on the graph. The voltage in the tiny terminal arbor branch[1] declines like a staircase of unevenly-spaced steps. Is the voltage falling most steeply in the boutons or in the tiny axon processes connecting the boutons?

## RECORD VOLTAGE-VS-TIME TRACES AT SELECTED POSITIONS ALONG THE AXON AND TERMINAL ARBOR BRANCH

### 1. *Bring up the Voltage-vs-Time graph*

This window will display recordings from eight (!) color-coded electrodes. The electrode positions are as follows:

- Four of the electrodes record from the myelinated portion of the axon at nodes 3 (red), 2 (green), 1 (blue), and 0 (black) (with node numbers decreasing in the direction of the nerve terminal).

- The fifth (brown) electrode is located in the middle of the heminode.

- The final three electrodes record from the first three boutons in the central terminal branch (branch[1]), and are color-coded as (bouton[1][0])(red), (bouton[1][1])(green), and (bouton[1][2])(blue).

### 2. *Questions about the Voltage-vs-Time traces*

- Why does the amplitude of the action potential <u>decrease as it approaches</u> the unmyelinated terminal arbor?

- Why does the action potential at the node closest to the heminode have a <u>double peak</u>?

- Why does the action potential suddenly increase in amplitude when it hits the <u>heminode</u>?

- What factors determine the <u>voltages in the branch</u> of the arbor?

## OBSERVE THE CURRENT PATTERNS IN A BRANCH OF THE TERMINAL ARBOR

It is difficult, if not impossible, to record membrane potentials from the tiny pre-synaptic terminals of NMJs in vertebrates. Using the "<u>loose patch</u>" technique, however, <u>Lindgren and Moore (1989)</u> were able to record currents from lizard presynaptic terminals and, using simulations, infer Na and K channel densities that could produce these currents. It was important that the parameters chosen allow a good match for all of the traces.

Here, you can reproduce their simulations and compare them to the recorded currents. We hope to illustrate the <u>process of matching</u> simulated traces to experimentally observed traces in order to gain insight into a problem.

### 1. *Open the Terminal Currents graph*

In this window you can plot the currents at various locations in the nerve terminal, color-coded to their label, starting with the heminode and proceeding through the boutons of the middle branch to its end.

## 2. *Examine the currents throughout the arbor*

Run the simulation. The only inward current is at the heminode; the remainder of the currents are outward, but of complex waveform.

## 3. *Compare the currents with the <u>published observations</u>*

The published records include a (labeled) stimulus artifact not present in the simulations of the tutorial. While the simulations are not a perfect match to the experimental data, the important point is that they give a good match for all five traces.

## 4. *Can you make a better match than the default values generate?*

If you are striving for a better match to the experimentally observed currents, the criterion for the match is that traces at the heminode, as well as at all of the boutons, fit the experimental data in time and amplitude.

- Call up the Heminode Parameters panel and the Bouton Parameters tray of panels to see the default values of the Na and K channel densities (conductances).

- Make changes to the values of the conductances in the Bouton Parameters panel and see how they change the current patterns. For any particular bouton, increase and decrease the Na channel density twofold, then do the same for the K channel density.

- Can a change in one bouton affect currents throughout the terminal, or does it only affect the currents in that bouton?

## EXPERIMENT WITH FACTORS AFFECTING INVASION OF THE PRESYNAPTIC ARBOR

When the axon becomes myelin-free at the terminal region, the situation seems similar to that in the Partial Demyelination tutorial, where the impulse failed to invade the bare axon. Clearly, invasion of the presynaptic arbor does not fail but demonstrates a robust design. What factors are important in invasion of the terminal?

## 1. *How important for invasion is the length of the last internode?*

In the Partial Demyelination tutorial, you observed that slightly <u>reducing the length</u> of the internode next to the bare axon supplied more longitudinal current to the unmyelinated portion and improved the chances that it would give an impulse. How important is the length of the last internode at the nerve terminal?

- **Bring up the Internode Lengths panel.**
  *Increase* the length of the last internode (Myelin[0]) by two or even three times. (Since you are increasing the length of the axon by doing this, the voltage change in the terminal branch will happen beyond the axes of the Voltage-vs-Space plots.) Look at the Voltage-vs-Time graph. What is the effect of such a large <u>change in the length of this internode</u> on the action potentials recorded in the heminode and in the boutons?

- **Return the internode to its default length.**

## 2. How important for invasion is the Na channel density in the heminode?

The heminode's Na conductance (0.6 S/cm$^2$) is five times that of the squid axon (0.12 S/cm$^2$). Does invasion of the terminal arbor depend on this value being so large? Divide this value by five so that it is the "normal" (squid axon) value and observe the results in the Voltage-vs-Time plot.

## 3. How important for invasion are the values of the Na conductances in the boutons?

The Na conductances in the boutons are higher than normal in all of the boutons. If you set them all to the squid axon value of 0.12 S/cm$^2$, what is the effect on invasion? What if you also set the Na conductance of the heminode to 0.12 S/cm$^2$? Click <u>here</u> for a discussion.

## 4. Invasion of the presynaptic terminal is robust, in contrast to the demyelinated axon

Nature has made sure that the action potential is able to invade the myelin-free presynaptic terminal of the NMJ despite the increased capacitive load it presents. The arbor branches are short, confining the entering current to flow across the membrane, thus depolarizing it. The amount of membrane in the arbor that must be depolarized is relatively small. Finally, the Na channel density is high, especially at the entrance to the arbor (the heminode), giving a large safety factor for the action potential.

## CONCLUSION

It should now be obvious that one reason the action potential can invade the arbor is because of the high density of Na channels, particularly at the heminode. The closed end of the arbor is also important.

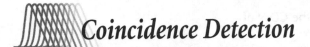# Coincidence Detection

## Achieving Temporal Precision in Integrating Synaptic Inputs

**Coincidence detection underlies integration in CNS neurons.**
Experiments of the past decade have led to a more sophisticated understanding of how inputs on CNS neurons interact over time and space. Previously, the firing of a neuron was thought to result from the summation of the synaptic inputs on the cell. But the current view is that the *relative timing*, or coincidence, of its inputs determines whether or not a neuron fires, and, consequently, how sharply tuned it is to the stimulus pattern it is designed to detect.

**The time period (window) over which inputs interact is crucial for tuning.**
Neurons of the auditory system that code frequency or localize sound provide well-understood examples of exquisite coincidence detection. These neurons have narrow "coincidence detection windows" (CDWs) that enable subthreshold EPSPs, arriving simultaneously, to sum and cause the cell to fire. Such neurons are sharply tuned to their stimulus, such as a particular frequency or particular sound location, because their narrow CDW prevents them from responding to asynchronous inputs. This tutorial focuses on mechanisms of achieving a narrow CDW, taking auditory neurons as the model.

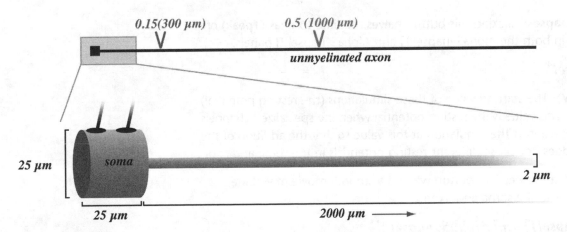

**The octopus cell of the mammalian cochlear nucleus provides the model for this tutorial.**
For simplicity, we have chosen to eliminate dendrites, which would provide capacitive load, as you have seen in the Site of Impulse Initiation tutorial. Nevertheless, much can be learned from experimenting with a simple system in which two synaptic inputs are placed directly on a soma attached to an unmyelinated axon. Myelination of the axon would be expected to cause the impulse to initiate at a point farther away from the soma, as in the Synaptic Integration tutorial.

**Goals of this Tutorial**
- To investigate how the insertion of special channels influences the CDW of an auditory neuron
- To explore whether faster synapses or higher temperatures significantly narrow the CDW in these neurons

## Start the Simulation

Click this button to bring up the panels and windows of the simulation.

Start the Simulation

## Description of the Panels and Windows Customized for this Tutorial

### 1. Panel & Graph Manager

- **Find Threshold for Synapse 1:** When this button is clicked, NEURON searches for the action potential threshold of the soma by gradually or iteratively adjusting the size of the synaptic conductance (gmax) at AlphaSynapse[1]. (The gmax of AlphaSynapse[2] must be set to zero.)

- **Add Ih and Klva:** Clicking this button adds these two channels to the soma (but not the axon).

- **Faster Synapses:** Clicking this button halves the time-to-peak (Tpeak) of the EPSPs in both the AlphaSynapse[1] and AlphaSynapse[2] panels.

### 2. Run Control

- **Reset (mV):** The starting value of these simulations (the resting potential) is –73 mV. This value is the resting potential when the specialized channels are added; we start the simulation at this value so that the addition of the channels does not cause different resting potentials in the soma and axon.

- **Reset & Run Movie:** This button will run a smooth movie of voltage versus space in the soma and axon.

### 3. AlphaSynapse[1] and AlphaSynapse[2]

These two panels control the attributes of the two EPSPs on the soma. When the simulation is launched, neither input is functional, as both conductances (gmax) are set to zero. You will set the value of these conductances during the experiments.

### 4. Graphs

- **Voltage vs Time, Soma:** This graph plots only the soma voltage versus time.

- **Voltage vs Time, Soma and Axon:** This graph plots voltage versus time in the soma (black trace) and in the 2000 μm-long axon at 300 μm (0.15) and at 1000 μm (0.5) from the soma.

- **Voltage vs Space, Soma and Axon:** The soma is positioned at the left end of this graph and the axon extends 2000 μm to the right, with recording electrodes positioned as described above. We include the axon in this tutorial because here is where the impulse often initiates.

## Experiments and Observations

### FIND THE DURATION OF THE CDW FOR A SOMA WITH TWO SUBTHRESHOLD EXCITATORY INPUTS

### 1. First, find the conductance increase that is just at threshold for triggering the action potential

- **Click the "Find Threshold 1" button in the P&G Manager.**
  When you click this button, NEURON will search for the threshold conductance and display its value in the "AlphaSynapse[1]" panel. Think of the simulator delivering pulses of neurotransmitter from the virtual presynaptic terminal at AlphaSynapse[1] onto the postsynaptic soma. The iterative pulses will be of concentrations above and below the threshold value until a concentration is found that is just at threshold.

- **If you Keep Lines in the Voltage-vs-Time graph, you can more easily track the process of finding the threshold.**
  You may find it interesting to repeat this process several times as sometimes NEURON approaches threshold from above and sometimes from below.

- **Where does the impulse initiate?**
  Does it <u>initiate</u> in the soma (or in the axon as in the <u>Site of Impulse Initiation</u> tutorial)?

### 2. Specify a conductance value for each subthreshold EPSP

To make a narrow CDW, you want the sum of the EPSPs to be *reliably above, but very near*, threshold. How large should their amplitudes be?

- **Choose the amplitude for each synaptic input.**

  - If each synaptic conductance were exactly half the threshold value, then their sum might—or might not—reach threshold and the postsynaptic soma would fire unreliably.

  - Should you set each synaptic conductance at 1% above the half-threshold value? In a simulation, this small increase above the half-threshold value should lead the EPSPs to sum reliably above threshold, but in reality, 1% would probably be too small to cover variability.

  - Here we arbitrarily choose 10%.

- **Calculate the value for the subthreshold synaptic conductances.**

  - You should have observed 0.04 μS for the threshold conductance caused by the neurotransmitter at this synapse.

  - 10% above threshold is 1.1 times 0.04 μS = 0.044 μS.

  - Half of 0.044 μS is 0.022 μS; this value will be the subthreshold gmax assigned to each synapse.

### 3. Now determine the CDW

- **Enter the conductance (gmax) value of 0.022 μS in each AlphaSynapse panel.**
  This is the value determined in the last step.

- **Delay the onset of AlphaSynapse[2] until this EPSP fails to sum with the first to evoke an action potential.**
  What is the <u>time difference</u> between the two synaptic inputs? This value is the CDW for a soma (with an axon attached and expressing only HH channels) when each EPSP is 10% above a half-threshold value at 6.3°C.

- **Reset the gmax of AlphaSynapse[2] to zero to prepare for the next threshold search.**

## SIMULATE AN AUDITORY NEURON BY ADDING SPECIALIZED CHANNELS TO THE SOMA

Two channel types, <u>Ih and Klva</u> conductances, are expressed selectively in certain auditory neurons. These channels lower the input resistance, and thus the time constant, of these neurons. The shorter time constant leads to a narrower CDW. Nature is clever in using these two channel types together to lower input resistance: Since opposing currents flow through the two channel types, the resting membrane potential remains stable.

### 1. Click the "Add Ih and Klva" button in the P&G Manager

- **The Ih and Klva conductances will be added to the soma.**

  - The Ih conductance (also called HCNO in the literature) begins to be activated at about −40 mV and is more strongly activated as the cell is hyperpolarized. Thus, it is partially activated at the resting potential and carries a steady inward current.

  - The Klva (low voltage activated K) conductance is activated at the resting potential and carries a steady outward current that balances the Ih inward current.

- **The changes appear in the Soma Parameters panel.**

  - In the Soma Parameters panel, the Ih and Klva conductances now have values. The Ih channel makes the membrane more excitable; the Klva channel reduces excitability.

### 2. Determine the CDW for the soma with these two channel types in its membrane

You will again determine the CDW by the same process as in the experiment above. But now the resting conductance of the cell is much higher. How will these changes affect the EPSPs, the site of impulse initiation, and the CDW?

- **Determine a subthreshold EPSP conductance value.**

  - Find the threshold for AlphaSynapse[1] as you did above. Before rushing on to determine the CDW, observe several interesting differences in the cell's response to the EPSP—consequences of having inserted the specialized channels:

> The first <u>difference</u> is in the amplitude and rate of rise of the EPSP in the soma necessary to generate a spike.

> The second difference is that now the impulse begins first in the axon and only later occurs in the soma. The time difference between the two action potentials can be as much as a millisecond, with the spike in the soma occurring when the EPSP's depolarization has returned almost to baseline. <u>Why is this</u>?

- **Now calculate the subthreshold conductance for each AlphaSynapse.**

  > Multiply the threshold value by 1.1, then set each synaptic conductance to half of the product.

- **Vary the onset of AlphaSynapse[2] to find the CDW when the soma includes the Ih and Klva channels**

  - How has the insertion of the two channels into the soma caused the <u>duration</u> of this CDW to change?

## WOULD INCREASING THE TEMPERATURE NARROW THE CDW APPRECIABLY?

As you have seen in previous tutorials, raising the temperature speeds channel kinetics, which leads to faster action potentials. Does raising the temperature narrow the CDW?

### 1. *Raise the temperature by 20°C to 26.3°C, leaving the specialized channels in the membrane*

Repeat the process of finding subthreshold synaptic conductances 10% above half-threshold. (Set AlphaSynapse[2] to 0, find threshold using AlphaSynapse[1], multiply this value by 1.1, divide by two, and enter this value into the conductance field of both synapse menus.) You will observe a smaller action potential in the soma since the normal HH channel densities <u>do not generate</u> a full-blown spike above about 16°C.

### 2. *Find the CDW at 26.3°C*

- You should find that the CDW has decreased to less than <u>half</u> of what it was at 6.3°C. Also, curiously, the spike in the soma diminishes in amplitude as the CDW widens and eventually fails altogether, although a full spike is elicited in the axon. An experimenter recording only from a soma might think that no impulse had been generated in this case!

- Although *NIA* is based on the HH channels found in squid axon and does not have the ability to simulate mammalian and avian temperatures and channels, you can imagine that higher temperatures would lead to even more narrowing of the CDW and thus greater and greater precision for neurons to detect the coincidence of inputs.

## CAN YOU FURTHER NARROW THE CDW BY DECREASING THE TIME TO PEAK OF THE SYNAPTIC CONDUCTANCE?

1. *Click the "Faster Synapses" button in the P&G Manager.*

   This action will halve the time-to-peak of each conductance. Leave the temperature at 26.3°C and keep the specialized channels in the membrane.

2. *Repeat the process of finding gmax <u>values</u> for the subthreshold synaptic inputs, then for the CDW.*

   How great an effect does this change have on the CDW? Is this one way in which the precision of coincidence detection can be improved in a neuronal circuit?

3. *Can the CDW be decreased further by decreasing the subthreshold gmax amplitudes?*

   By how much can you narrow the CDW if you reduce the percent by which each gmax is above half-threshold? Remember that in real cells, working with such marginal inputs risks compromising reliability because of the variability of the amplitudes of synaptic events.

# *"Voltage Clamping" Intact Cells*

## Looking at the Action Behind the Scenes

**Simulations reveal what is actually happening when "voltage clamping" with a single electrode.**
In contrast to the experimental display of voltages and currents with an electrode located in a cell body, the simulations in this tutorial display the voltages throughout the cell in both space and time. This information is simply beyond current experimental possibilities. The graphs here will allow you to see any degradations of voltage control everywhere in the modeled neuron and realize that there could be much more going on than you observe experimentally. If you end up with a sense of "Caveat Clamper," the goals of the exercises here will have been met.

**Currents flowing *within* the neuron complicate attempts to voltage clamp whole cells.**
To understand how an intact neuron functions, you might wish to characterize its voltage- and synaptically-gated currents. But is the voltage across this membrane the actual value set with the clamp? Whether you are interested in channels in the soma, the dendrites, or the synaptic terminals, how do you know if your currents are actually flowing through those channels and not flowing from some other portion of the cell?

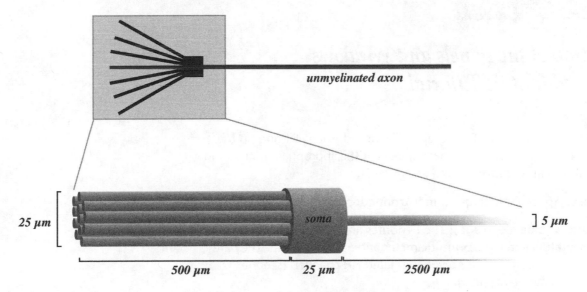

**Here you will experiment with clamping the soma of the simplest possible neuron.**
In the Voltage Clamping a Patch tutorial, by definition, the voltage was uniform at every point in the membrane, an ideal situation. Here, you can experiment with clamping the soma of the neuron in the Site of Impulse Initiation tutorial. You will see how moving from a patch to more complex

geometry can affect your recorded currents. You can also experiment with the <u>series resistance</u> of the electrode, which can dramatically affect voltage clamp currents.

**Clamping the soma of an intact neuron is far different from clamping a patch.**

Voltage clamping a patch leads to interpretable results. Consequently the "patch clampers" have pulled patches off dendrites and somata of CNS neurons, <u>for example</u>, to characterize the voltage-gated channels in those locations. Voltage clamp records from a whole cell, in contrast, must be interpreted with great caution. But whole cell experiments are often necessary. What if the cell must be intact because the currents are synaptic or are the result of intracellular signaling?

**Goals of this Tutorial**

- To observe how the capacitance of the (passive) dendritic tree affects currents and voltage steps in a "voltage clamped" soma
- To observe how longitudinal currents flowing from the axon or dendrites distort currents one thinks are flowing across the soma's membrane in a "clamped" soma
- To observe how the resistance of the electrode can degrade the control of the voltage by the clamp

# Start the Simulation

Click this button to bring up the panels and windows of the simulation.

> **Start the Simulation**

# Description of the Panels and Windows Customized for this Tutorial

## 1. The graphs

At first, only the Current-vs-Time graph is launched. You will bring up the Voltage-vs-Time and Voltage-vs-Space graphs at the appropriate moment in the tutorial using the buttons in the P&G Manager.

- **Voltage vs Space (see diagram in Introduction)**

  ▪ **Dendrites (blue electrode):** The dendrites are "collapsed" into a representational tree of 25 μm diameter and 500 μm length. They are passive; that is, they have no voltage-gated HH channels (see the Dendrite Parameters panel).

  ▪ **Soma (red electrode):** The soma, here 25 μm by 25 μm, contains HH Na and K channels at their default density (see the Soma Parameters panel).

  ▪ **Axon (black electrode):** The axon, 5 μm in diameter and 2500 μm in length, is unmyelinated and contains default HH channels (see Axon Parameters Panel). The electrode is positioned one-tenth of the way from the soma to the axon's far end.

### 2. Stimulus Control, <u>Single Electrode Voltage Clamp</u>

This version of the Stimulus Control panel uses a single electrode both to clamp the voltage and record the current, the normal patch clamp situation (and used for sharp electrodes as well). The values of the Conditioning, Command (Testing), and Return pulses are displayed as in the <u>Voltage Clamping a Patch</u> tutorial and are set by default at –65, –40, and –65 mV.

The electrode resistance is specified in the field associated with the "Rs, Mohm" button.

## Experiments and Observations

### CLAMP THE SOMA WITH AN IDEAL, LOW-RESISTANCE ELECTRODE AND MEASURE THE RESULTING CURRENT

The resistance of the electrode, "Rs, Mohm" in the Stimulus Control panel, is set at a very low "ideal" default value, 0.01 Mohm (Rs would be zero for a truly ideal voltage clamp). At this value, the electrode resistance should not distort your observations of voltage and current.

### 1. Run the simulation and examine the current trace

The current trace may seem complicated. To simplify it, remember that the total membrane current has two components: the capacitive current, Icap; and the ionic current, Iionic, flowing through the HH channels.

- **Icap**
  Notice that the instantaneous, large, brief surge of outward current at the beginning of the pulse is essentially equal in amplitude and time course to the inward current surge following the end of the pulse. This current, Icap, charges and discharges the membrane capacitance. The lower the electrode resistance, the higher this current and the more quickly the capacitance is charged and discharged. The ideal situation is for Icap to cease before the ionic (Na and K) currents begin so that it does not distort them.

  The amplitude of Icap can give an approximate measure of the <u>electrode resistance</u>.

- **Ionic current**
  Following the Icap is first an inward current, then an outward current. A reasonable guess is that you are observing the inward sodium current (INa) and the outward K current (IK).

- **Questions about the current:**
  Why is there an inflection on the rising phase of the inward current? Is the Icap interfering? Or is this distortion perhaps due to axial (longitudinal) current flowing into the soma from the dendrites or the axon? If so, perhaps the current you are measuring is not simply the current across the membrane of the soma that you might think you are measuring. The experiments below should give some insight.

### 2. Bring up the Voltage-vs-Time and Voltage-vs-Space graphs to observe the voltage change in the dendrites and axon

Simulations allow you, while clamping the soma, to record the voltage in parts of the neuron that would commonly be inaccessible in a real experiment.

In the Voltage-vs-Time panel, there are now four traces to follow:

- **The command voltage (brown trace)**

- **The soma voltage (red trace)**
  In this case, because the electrode resistance is negligible, the voltage in the soma tracks the command voltage perfectly so the red and brown traces overlay each other. Below you will learn that this is the ideal situation and is only rarely experienced in real experiments.

- **The dendritic voltage (blue trace)**
  Note that the voltage in the dendrites lags the command voltage slightly. You can change dendritic parameters to check your reasoning about why this happens.

- **The axon voltage (black trace)**
  Clearly the axon gives an action potential. Notice where it is initiated.

- **Questions about the voltage changes you are observing:**

  - Why does the voltage in the dendrites change more slowly than the voltage in the soma?

  - Why doesn't the electrode control the voltage in the axon as well as in the soma?

  - After initiation in the axon, why doesn't the action potential conduct backwards into the soma?

- **Keep Lines in the current trace for comparing these observations with those in the following experiments.**

## HOW DOES BLOCKING THE AXONAL CHANNELS AFFECT SOMA CURRENTS?

Did longitudinal current, flowing from the axon's action potential towards the soma, add to the current actually flowing through the soma's membrane? Any longitudinal current from the axon would have produced a misleading distortion in the current you observed.

With the NEURON simulator you can test the hypothesis that longitudinal currents from the axon contributed to your measured currents by using TTX and TEA to block the Na and K currents individually in the axon but not the soma. In real experiments, it is rare to be able to isolate cell domains pharmacologically, although certain preparations lend themselves to it (for example, the barnacle photoreceptor studied by one of the authors of *NIA*).

### 1. *Put TTX on the axon*

The axon is giving an action potential. By blocking it with TTX, will you change the current observed in the soma?

- **Set the Na channel density in the axon to zero and run the simulation.**
  Doing so should block the generation of a spike in the axon. Does it change the current recorded in the soma?

- **Questions about the current in the soma when TTX blocks Na channels in the axon:**

- What is the difference in the inward ionic (Na) current between the two situations? Can the TTX experiment help explain the inflection in the rising phase of the somatic inward current when the axon was permitted to give an action potential?

- If you were to observe an inflection of the rising phase of an inward current in a real experiment on a cell, should you not suspect problems with voltage nonuniformity?

- **Examine the voltage trace in the axon in TTX.**
  Can you explain its shape? If not, perhaps the next experiment will help.

## 2. *Add TEA, a K channel blocker, to the TTX already on the axon*

Before doing the experiment, think: Do you expect that adding TEA to the axon will cause a further change in the current recorded in the soma? What sort of change?

- **Set both the Na and K channel densities in the axon to zero.**
  Run the simulation.

- Question:

  - What is the value of the <u>voltage</u> plateau in the axon during the clamp step with the axon bathed in TTX and TEA? Why is it not at the same value as the voltage in the soma? Hint: Look at the Voltage-vs-Space plot and stop the simulation during the pulse.

- **Return the axonal conductances to their default settings.**

## EXPERIMENT WITH LIGATING FIRST THE AXON, THEN THE DENDRITIC TREE

The experiments above probably revealed that drugs cannot completely isolate one part of a cell (the axon) from another (the soma). How can the active axon or the passive dendrites be isolated from the soma so as to observe the true somatic current? In actual experiments it is sometimes possible to ligate axons but almost impossible to ligate dendrites. On the computer, however, one can ligate either axon, dendrites, or both, to achieve isolation—and possible insight.

## 1. *Ligate the axon*

- **Set the diameter of the axon to zero and run the simulation.**
  When you enter zero, NEURON will set the diameter to an infinitesimally small value.

- **Does ligating the axon give the same result as blocking its channels?**

## 2. *Restore the diameter of the axon and ligate the dendrites*

Because the axon is now free again to give an action potential, the longitudinal current from the axon will once again contribute to the current recorded in the soma. But has ligating the dendrites changed the current you record in the default situation (no ligations or drugs)? Has it changed Icap, Iionic (inward and outward), or all of the above, and can you explain any change?

- **What, then, is the true value of the inward current in the soma?**
  To observe the true value of the inward current through somatic channels,

you probably have realized that you must ligate both axon and dendrites. We hope these simulations help you evaluate published voltage clamp records involving whole cells.

- **Restore the diameters of the dendrites and axon to their default values.**

## CHANGE THE RESISTANCE OF THE ELECTRODE

The patch clamp technique has greatly improved the ability of electrodes to pass current into cells by allowing pipettes to be fatter in bore at the tip. Nevertheless, pipettes are still long, skinny glass conduits and the conducting medium with which they are filled has resistance. This "series resistance" can distort clamp currents.

### 1. Mimic a typical whole-cell patch experiment by setting Rs to 0.1 Mohm

Before running the simulation, run and save the default "ideal" simulation (Rs = 0.01 Mohm) in order to compare voltages and currents for the two pipette values. Also, try to predict what will happen to the voltage and current in the soma, dendrites, and axon when you increase pipette resistance.

- **What is happening to the voltage in the three regions of the cell when Rs is increased?**
  Things are now rather complicated: The voltage changes in all three regions are different when the electrode resistance increases. Can you explain what is taking place?

- **What is happening to the current in the soma?**
  The amplitudes and time courses of both Icap and the inward Na current have changed. Can you explain why? Everyone likes to publish records of big currents but perhaps big currents are not necessarily a good thing!

### 2. Increase Rs by another order of magnitude (from 0.1 to 1 Mohm)

You are now progressing from an ideal clamp (Rs = 0.01 Mohm) through a more typical clamp (Rs = 0.1 Mohm) to an out-of-control clamp (Rs = 1 Mohm).

- **Now, what a disaster! What is happening to the voltage in the three regions of the cell?**
  The electrode now cannot pass enough current to clamp the soma at the commanded value. Clearly the voltage in the soma is being governed by the cell's voltage-gated channels and not by the clamp amplifier. But why do we see what looks like a small action potential in the "passive" dendrites? How can you explain this observation?

- **Questions about the voltage and current traces in the out-of-control clamp (Rs = 1 Mohm):**

  - Explain the dramatic change in Icap in the soma. Look carefully at Icap. What has happened to its amplitude? To its time course?

  - Explain the dramatic change in the inward Na current in the soma. Why is the inward current now smaller? Why is it so delayed? What is the source of this current?

### 3. *How does dendritic ligation affect the results in an out-of-control clamp?*

The voltage change in the dendrites is a dramatic consequence of this poor clamp. How are the dendrites affecting the voltage and current in the soma, and the voltage in the axon? Remove them and find out.

- **Compare simulations with and without the dendrites ligated (Rs = 1 Mohm).**
  This experiment should give you an increased awareness of the capacitive load placed on a cell soma by its dendritic tree. We hope the set of experiments in this tutorial also makes you approach voltage clamp observations in cells with informed caution.